THE PILL,
JOHN ROCK,
AND THE CHURCH

THE PILL,
JOHN ROCK,
AND THE CHURCH

The Biography of a Revolution

by Loretta McLaughlin

Little, Brown and Company   Boston • Toronto

15.95 BJT 1-18-83

FIRST EDITION

Library of Congress Cataloging in Publication Data

McLaughlin, Loretta.
    The pill, John Rock, and the church.

    Includes index.
        1. Oral contraceptives — United States — History.
    2. Oral contraceptives — Religious aspects — Catholic
    Church. 3. Rock, John Charles, 1890-
    4. Gynecologists — United States — Biography.
    5. Medical research personnel — United States — Biog-
    raphy. I. Title.
    RG137.5.M38   1982   613.9′432′0924   [B]   82-16187
    ISBN 0-316-56095-2

*The author is grateful to the following publishers to quote
material as noted:*

AP Newsfeatures for permission to quote from the August
4, 1944 wire story by Howard Blakeslee on Test Tube Fertilization.

Harvard University Press for excerpts from *Contraception:
A History of the Development of the Doctrine by Catholic
Theologians* by John Noonan. Reprinted by permission.

MV
Designed by Dale Cotton

*Published simultaneously in Canada
by Little, Brown & Company (Canada) Limited*

PRINTED IN THE UNITED STATES OF AMERICA

To my very dear friend, James Peter Becker

ACKNOWLEDGMENTS

I WANT to thank everyone who helped me with this book.

Foremost is Richard McDonough, my editor at Little, Brown, who from beginning to end saw what the book should be and held me to it.

I also am grateful to Richard Wolfe, curator of the Rare Books Collection at Countway Medical Library, who trusted me with papers and files not yet catalogued and bent the rules a bit so that I could be comfortable while I went through them.

James King, vice-president for communications, and his assistant Janet Blowney of Brigham and Women's Hospital extended their help many times in a multitude of ways — always most graciously.

I also appreciate the generosity of the news staff at the *Boston Pilot* in permitting me to use their news files.

At the *Boston Globe* my colleagues James Franklin, religion editor, and George Collins, former head librarian and now director of the Boston Globe Foundation, let me use them as sounding boards and also located vital materials and books for me. *Boston Globe* editor Tom Winship gave real encouragement when it was much needed.

There are many others to whom I am indebted, particularly those who, through interviews, filled in the missing pieces. They really made the book possible.

I would like to commend my friends who were — to borrow John Rock's favorite expression — so *tolerant* of my preoccupation with the book; especially Rosanne Ring and Margaret Murphy who sometimes rode along with me on long drives to interviews or out-of-the-way libraries, and who found out-of-print books for me. I would also like to thank my friends Dr. Kenneth Bird and Amy Selwyn not only for spotting special references for me but also for never doubting that I would finish the book.

My children, Ruth, Mark and Neil, deserve medals for their patience and understanding and even more for their unflagging support. They cheered me on at every turn.

I also appreciate the permission granted by Professor John T. Noonan, Jr. and by Harvard University Press for use of excerpts from his great reference work: *Contraception, A History of Its Treatment by the Catholic Theologians and Canonists.*

My ultimate thanks, however, goes to Jim Becker, who was first editor throughout.

CONTENTS

PROLOGUE

JOHN ROCK belongs now and forever to that select company of mortals who profoundly changed the world.

He did it in a most remarkable way, at one and the same time on the most intimate personal terms and on a universal scale. Moreover, he did it knowingly.

"My first job was to preserve the family," he muses, "and after that, the Family of Man."

To do it, he placed within the reach of men and women everywhere, whose lives were virtually held hostage by the threat of constant pregnancy, a wholly new means for their deliverance.

He gave them "the pill," a simple-to-use and utterly effective contraceptive, the greatest advance in contraceptive research in history and the first medicine ever destined for a purely social, rather than a therapeutic, purpose.

His foremost concern was the family and the creation of a means to let husband and wife love and mate without fear that the sexual expression of their love would produce one child after another willy-nilly; children they were in no position to raise.

He understood, as few did at the time, that a robust and vigorous sex life made for a good marriage. Sexual closeness, he was certain, was the mortar that bonded couples together firmly enough to withstand the strain of raising children well.

Rock's extraordinary little pill, however, carried far greater potential than safeguarding against unwanted pregnancy during what he called "the joyful fulfillment" of the marital act.

To a degree never before envisioned, it set men and women free sexually. And, as it turned out, it did so to an extent that far exceeded Rock's original intentions. The pill became a cornerstone of the sexual revolution that swept the industrialized countries of the world from the mid-1960s on.

The pill also did much to legitimize the rightful study and understanding of human sexuality, long ignored by serious, albeit sanctimonious, scientists. Its acceptance also stimulated the search for other improved forms of contraception, most notably, the IUD, or intrauterine device. Further, the availability of the pill, with its assurance that pregnancies could be reliably planned and timed, strongly abetted the women's movement, opening the way for prolonged academic study without interruption and for career commitment.

Most of all, however, the pill provided the first real hope that the new menace in the world, runaway population growth, could be controlled. In time, this became Rock's all-pervasive concern.

He became convinced that there was no choice, no alternative, except to grapple head on with "the first *world* problem in history and by far the most perilous to mankind," that of overpopulation. Time was running out, if huge-scale disaster — massive starvation and social mayhem — were to be avoided.

Mankind's unbridled fecundity, as he saw it, posed a greater threat than the nuclear bomb. "The human species must set limits on its ratio of reproduction or allow the general welfare to perish in a savage battle for survival," he held. The pill, he believed, offered the first meaningful new prospect that somehow the gathering whirlwind of excessive population could be tamed.

To provide womankind with the pill was one monumental step, but to convince the world of the rightness of its use was another, and far more difficult, one. Even to begin to achieve the larger end, Rock had to rally support against age-old societal and religious resistance.

It fell to Rock to become the pill's foremost spokesman, and to become the single, most effective voice of conscience from the laity that would dare to challenge the last great bastion of opposition to birth control — that of his own, beloved Roman Catholic Church.

It is in those roles, as champion of the pill and challenger to the Church, that Rock's greatness looms largest, transcending even the pivotal role he played in uncovering the contraceptive power of the pill.

THE PILL,
JOHN ROCK,
AND THE CHURCH

1

PREPARATION FOR LIFE

THE population of the world had not yet crept past the 1.5 billion mark in 1890, but the population bomb was already beginning to tick. It was a sound that John Rock would one day hear and heed. He would, together with reproductive biologists Gregory Pincus and Min-Chueh Chang, forge the key to the regulation of female fertility and do so in the full ironic light of his religious commitment and his lifetime search for solutions to infertility. In time, too, gathering world forces would single out John Rock, beyond any other, to contend with the unbending stance of the Roman Catholic Church on birth control. It would become Rock's destiny to introduce the new way to prevent unwanted pregnancy to society and to challenge the Church of Rome — along with the rest of the world — to accept it.

On March 24 of that year John Rock was born, some twenty minutes ahead of his twin sister Ellen.

Although of no concern whatever to the Rock family of Marlborough, Massachusetts at the time, an extraordinary change was taking place in some of the highly Catholic countries of Western Europe, most notably France and Belgium. The birthrate was beginning to decline. The mode of contraception most responsible for this phenomenon was *coitus interruptus,* premature withdrawal; the biblical sin of onanism, the deliberate spilling of the male "seed" outside the female receptacle.

Contrary to what might be expected, the attitude of the Catholic hierarchy toward such contraceptive acts by married couples was surprisingly tolerant. Vatican authorities observed that priests would be wise to "be silent, unless asked," about the marital practices of confessors. Though stricter theological opinions were voiced occasionally, the Church was content for the time to leave the issues of marital sex and birth control to the dictates of parish clergy. All of this was far removed from the first generation of Rocks to be born in their new country — America.

John Rock is the namesake of his grandfather, a native of the township of Armagh, County Armagh, just north of the embattled boundary that now separates Northern Ireland from the Republic of Ireland. He immigrated to Boston in the wake of the lethal potato famine that decimated the Irish in the mid-1800s and drove millions of them to the United States.

The founding father Rock organized the passage for a boatload of Irish immigrants, half-starved from the potato famine, to this country, according to the family records. He supported himself as a tailor. And as did many Irish immigrants of the era, he put every penny not required for the family's support into land.

Grandfather Rock settled in the town of Marlborough, whose small mills and huge waterworks aside the reservoir attracted many of the newly arrived Irish. Others readily took to the farms or set up shop as tradesmen, as the elder Rock did. Located nearer to Worcester in central Massachusetts than to Boston on the coast, the town could scarcely be distinguished from dozens of others, appealing primarily for its untrammeled openness and simple day-to-day life. It was heavily Catholic in numbers but governed and outclassed by a Protestant gentry and the relatively new Yankee minor industrialists, whose more mannered style from the outset held great fascination for young John Rock.

"My sainted mother was Ann Jane Murphy and my father — not so sainted — was Frank Sylvester Rock," John noted. When Grandfather Rock died, however, Frank had to leave high school and go to work immediately with his older brother, John, to try to pay off the mortgages left by their land-hungry father. In his insatiable desire for property, he had bought land and buildings all over town with a minimum downpayment on each one.

The two brothers had that canny talent that it is said the Irish abound in, an unsquelchable zest for life with which they handily combined business and pleasure. In the process they always managed to make just enough money more than was essential, to indulge their personal interests. John Rock was to be the same.

First, the Rock brothers opened a drugstore at what was dubbed by the townies Rock's Corner. The brothers were known, not unexpectedly, to sell a little "strong" medicine in the back room. Recognizing the better profit in liquor, they next opened a saloon at Monument Square, farther up on Main Street in the then embryonic business district of Marlborough. That proved so successful, they built the Rock building next door and incorporated within it a substantial theater, replete with an ingenious movable stage for traveling vaudeville and repertory companies. Eventually, the theater became one of the early moving picture houses. Rock thought his father never really had much taste for the saloon business, but "the two brothers were so saddled with bills inherited from their father, they needed to make some money fast, you see." Rock acquired a taste for the essence of all three of the brothers' early enterprises: medicine, liquor, and the dramatic arts.

On his own, Frank Rock built and operated an excellent racetrack on a tract of his father's mortgaged land, dabbled in breeding race horses, and developed a small but creditable stable. Both for fun and profit, he also organized the Marlborough town baseball team, which played in a local semi-pro circuit. A wonderfully personable man, Frank Rock loved male sociability and the good life, characteristics that John fully shared. The father also reveled in innocent gambling, card-playing with the "boys" at the firehouse, some manly drinking, and his favorite sports, horse-racing and baseball. Like many other first-generation Irish, Frank Rock wanted his children to love their God, their Church, and their country and to revere their mother, his wife, as he surely did. Ann Jane Murphy wanted more: she wanted her children to have the formal education she and her husband had been denied. At home, she would make sure the children would be fully schooled in the social graces, which she considered of equal importance. Typical of the generation, Rock's father ran the external family affairs and his mother, the household.

What Rock remembered most tenderly, however, was that "they got along beautifully together. They were very, very close." His parent's devotion to one another was a model for Rock's own marriage later. His parents were equals in their own spheres, strong and respectful of one another's territory, but delighting in each other's company.

For their era Frank and Ann Rock were remarkably permissive parents; another model Rock was to adopt. They were not narrow, restrictive, or punitive as were many of the working-class Irish back then. Perhaps their economic freedom largely accounted for the freedom they granted their children. There was no need to be harsh. They were conscious, too, that their newfound prosperity permitted them to emulate more closely the established genteel Protestants in town whose children were spared menial occupations.

In the Rock household, the emphasis was on fundamental principles — faith, honor, loyalty, and deep moral values. These were the guiding lights, taught by the Church and practiced at home. So long as those guidelines were followed, then there was room for the rewards of pleasure and leisure. The Rocks were enormously proud, just as they were gutsy and quick-witted, full of good humor and a sense of their own worth.

The family lived in one of the properties acquired by Grandfather Rock on upper Main Street: a handsome, roomy, sturdily built and finely furnished homestead, but nonetheless a two-family duplex. It was always planned that one day they would occupy the whole house, but they were mindful of the security provided by rental income, especially when, as during Prohibition, money was tight.

It was here that the Rock twins, John and Ellen, were born, the youngest of five children. Charles (Charlie) was the eldest by six years, followed by Henry (Harry) and Mary (Maisie). Interestingly, all of Rock's mother's pregnancies, in a time preceding sophistication about child-spacing, occurred two years apart.

Life was exceptionally sedate for young John Rock, far more so than for his older brothers, who were rugged sports enthusiasts like their father. In many respects, the family style was toney for the times, given to those somewhat arch amenities later characterized as "high" Irish. They dined formally, cherished the finery of good china, crystal, and silver, heavy linens and thick rugs, the household appurtenances that bespoke of quality and correctness. Until Prohibition put a crimp in the family income, they had household help, a maid and a cook and, when the children were babies, a nursery woman.

Until he was twelve or more years old, John's constant companion and closest friend was his twin, Nell. His closeness to her indelibly marked his life, making him sensitive as few medical men were to the medical problems and feelings of women. Until they were five or six years old, they were bathed together, fed together, and slept in the same room. John far preferred her company to that of the "vulgar, bad-mannered boys" especially the Irish Catholic boys from the working-class families in the lower end of town with whom his brothers chummed, played football and baseball, and boxed. John enjoyed the girls' pursuits, playing house and dolls and skipping rope. Similarly to John D. Rockefeller, Jr., John Rock also learned to crochet and sew a little,* even attending one sewing class with Nell to his brothers' horror. His mother, however, sided with John, letting him go along if it was what he wanted to do. His girlish preferences, however, earned him the name "Sissy" Rock and account for some of what he called the "sissified mannerisms" that persisted through his life. His older brothers were really quite "tolerant" of his ways, tolerant being his favorite word to describe "how everyone has always put up with me."

On one occasion, however, Charlie lost his temper, Rock recalled. "Our parents were in Florida. Nell and I were about five years old and we were putting on one of our 'shows,' something we often did to entertain ourselves. We had double doors in the dining room through which we opened our act. Well, the highlight of this skit, in which we were pretending we were going swimming, was to expose our genitals. I suppose we knew it was a bit naughty, but thought it a splendid joke. I still remember Charlie slam-banging me for it."

It didn't, however, dampen his interest in performing. He and Nell learned to play the piano and became members of a local musical group fancily named the Orpheus Club that met in the Marlborough press club in Pythian Hall, another of his father's buildings. The club also introduced him to the practice of exclusivity, which he indulged extensively as an adult with memberships in some of Boston's restricted social clubs. Rock, admittedly a snob of sorts even as a child, gave in to the girls "to let in some boys that I wouldn't have, had I had the final say."

Later in life he chose to attribute his harmless childhood snobbishness to an inborn sensitivity: "I have always felt more comfortable with people who were superior to me — in ability. It wasn't an economic thing, not because they were richer or of social position, it was a matter of style, dress, conversation and cultural interests. But it's true, nonetheless, from the time I was in the first grade in Marlborough, I enjoyed the superior kids. Preferred their company. I was put off, still am, by crudeness. I feel it has affected my life for the good." His own children saw it less as snobbishness than "an absence of tolerance for stupidity. He had absolutely none."

* And even more like Texas heart surgeon Michael DeBakey, who as a youngster knotted the threads for his seamstress mother. Rock's penchant for sewing and other hand skills requiring great finger dexterity, such as piano playing, were to stand him in excellent stead later in life as a surgeon.

His aversion to boyish horseplay made for an unusual degree of isolation as he was growing up. "My father deprecated my isolation, my isolating of myself. Rugged, masculine boys didn't do that." Rock's father got on better with Charlie and Harry, than with John. They were older and nearer to him in his manly interests. John tried desperately to join their circle, unsuccessfully. He tried to memorize baseball scores so he could understand what they were talking about, but it wasn't in him. John and his father felt no lesser love for one another, however, and found ways to express that affection on their own terms: "I was always the one who would row him around the lake when he wanted to troll for bass. And when I developed pimples as an adolescent it was father who took me to his osteopath to see what could be done. The doctor told me I should take enemas. I asked what those were and he said soap and water. Naïvely, I protested that I couldn't swallow that and he explained, 'Oh, no, you put it in the other end.' Father roared."

He found great comfort and joy in his Catholicism; out of it came a profoundly formed conscience. He steeped himself in Catholic teachings, reading far more extensively than most of its practitioners ever do. The depth of his interest, knowledge, and commitment to his faith was to give him great strength in later years.

Even as a youth, he was the most religious member of the family. "Mother wasn't overly religious. Oh, she went to mass on Sundays and we said the rosary as a family every night during Lent. Even my father would come in sometimes and kneel down," Rock laughed, "that is if he happened to be home. I, on the other hand, was incredibly religious growing up." He became a daily communicant as a teenager at his parish church, the Immaculate Conception, in Marlborough, and for that reason, perhaps, often went out of his way to attend the church in Boston by the same name in later years. While by choice many of his teenage friends were Protestant boys (he would always be comfortable in Protestant company), whom he found more socially acceptable, he never wished he was one of them. Rather, he tried to enlighten them about Catholicism, "to show them what a gift it was. I'd take them to mass with me and to hear missionary priests."

In a daily journal he kept from the time he was a young schoolboy, one entry, on November 8, 1908, when he was eighteen years old, notes a rare, serious conversation with his father about philosophy, and "ethical" subjects. "I sympathize with my mother's concern about my father's lack of Catholicity," he wrote. "Once or twice I attempted to make an impression on him as concerned adhering to church rules, eating fish on Friday, telling him how and why and so on." Rock was later to comment about his father, "He was very tolerant about such matters, but not very impressed."

When Rock made up his mind that he wanted to leave Marlborough High School after his first year and switch to the new High School of Commerce in Boston, his father and mother approved the idea without hesitation. It was an adventurous move in 1906 for a young man to consider going to high school thirty-five miles from home. Rock had heard about Commerce High from friends at Lakeside, a summer colony at nearby Lake Boone in Hudson, where the Rock family summered. He thought they were "far superior to the gang at Marlborough High," and so, of course, he wanted to join them. Rock's parents arranged for John to board during the week with Delia and Tom Flynn in Boston's Back Bay. Tom Flynn was an old friend of Rock's father and a fellow entrepreneur in the liquor business. John got along famously with Tom, but didn't like Delia at all. In his estimation, "she was a cheapie." He liked her even less, when a decade later, following the death of her husband and Rock's mother, she became his stepmother.

After a month with the Flynns, Rock had had enough. On the pretext of packing for a weekend at home, he took everything, his clothes, family pictures, books, and toilet articles, and left. "I checked into the Hotel Clarendon" in Boston's Back Bay, he recalled, "and I hadn't been there an hour when Delia called to say, 'What's going on? Everything is gone.' " He countered with a touch of the decisiveness he would display later in his life, "Yes, and I have, too." He contacted a high school friend who had a room on Gainsborough Street and who got Rock lodging in the same boardinghouse. "My father came in to Boston immediately and took the Flynns and me to the theater to smooth things over. He gave me an extra ten dollars for fear I'd need it and that was all there was to it. He trusted me to be on my own. Why wouldn't he? I was a young man of the world, well able to take care of myself. He knew I wouldn't get in to any trouble and I didn't."

Actually, the move to Commerce High was of great significance in Rock's growing up. He discovered the elation of attending a school he liked, the intimacy of small classes, the excitement of studies that interested him and the camaraderie of an all-boys school. Suddenly, his latent interest in sports flowered and for the first time he enthusiastically joined in. He qualified for the running and swimming teams and became president of the school athletic association. He was popular at last with his peers in manly activities.

The High School of Commerce in Boston was a new venture in edu-

cation at the turn of the century. It was the brainchild of Frederick
Fish, a Boston corporate lawyer, and the Filene brothers, who not
only founded one of the city's most successful clothing and household
goods stores, but originated the concept of the bargain basement. They
were backed by a group of businessmen, including bank presidents and
the publishers of the city's two major newspapers, the *Herald Traveler*
and *Boston Globe*. Beyond the classically oriented Boston Public Latin
School and English High, these men thought Boston should have a
special high school to prepare young men for business careers. They
used the Harvard Graduate School of Business Administration as their
inspiration and ambitiously attempted to offer similar courses on a
slightly less erudite plane.

Rock "did very well there." He began to develop a competitive spirit
and in his senior year won an essay contest for which the prize was a
summer trip to South America. To the amusement of those who would
know his poor business habits later, he was very enamored of the idea
of going into business "and becoming a great businessman."

The world of business looked promising indeed to John Rock when
he graduated from the High School of Commerce in 1909, but he still
had no definite career in mind. His South America prize unexpectedly
paid off, however. The United Fruit Company hired him to work as a
timekeeper on one of its banana plantations in Guatemala. Within a
few months, he was promoted to manager of a six-mile-long farm. It
was there that he first saw the abuse of farm workers, Negroes and
native Indians, and the squalor of their lives. At that point, he was not
stirred by any revolutionary ideas of rescuing them, but the memory of
their misery stayed with him. Although Rock thought he was doing a
good job, he was fired at the end of nine months, "the normal gestation
period, a matter I have never understood. I can only attribute my loss
of that job to the inability of the United Fruit officials to realize what
a prize I was. Really, of course, I knew very little about what I was
doing."

Nonetheless, it was an eye-opening experience for a twenty-year-old.
Nothing in his orderly and comfortable earlier life had prepared him
for the Guatemalan banana camp. The cheapness of human life for the
workers was indelibly imprinted in his mind, particularly as it existed
in utter contrast to the wealth of the owners and aristocracy. He knew
from firsthand observation what medical colleagues from Central and
South America were talking about later: young men, old before their
time, shackled by lack of education and locked away from escape by

the responsibility of early marriage and large families. He took their example away with him. At the same time he started to study Spanish, a pasttime he continued throughout life. He also acquired a taste for fineries from other countries. That taste was sparked by a highborn Buenos Aires lady who "befriended" him. He came home with a fur rug and mantillas of Spanish lace, purchases his father considered foolishly extravagant and eventually had to pay for.

He next got a job with the engineering firm of Stone & Webster in their Woonsocket, Rhode Island, offices. "There I was equally ill-fitted for the work as cashier and general consultant to four of their companies with an office staff of four or five clerks. That went on for another nine-month gestation period until one day they discovered that I had a cash drawer full of quarters and a $100 check that I hadn't accounted for. That was the end of that." In all his life, he never overcame this casual attitude toward money.

This time the job loss really gave Rock cause for worry. His honesty had been questioned — though the matter was all straightened out later — and his record for holding a job was poor. Rock's "guardian angel was on the job, though," because he returned home in no disgrace. But the time for serious stock-taking had unquestionably come. Rock decided he wasn't suited for business after all and that he'd better go to college to try to learn something worthwhile. At just that time, Harvard College had relaxed its rules for admissions. Instead of having to take tests in twenty subjects, four would suffice. Rock, with the congenial help of a girlfriend who was a schoolteacher, studied German and French and brushed up on geometry. He passed the entrance exams, in part because "my guardian angel hadn't given up on me yet."

Rock was ecstatic and so was his family. His father happily assumed responsibility for the tuition, then $300 a year (and only $600, later, for medical school), plus an allowance. Rock's brother Charlie cautioned him not to be a bookworm, but to get out and meet people and socialize, advice that Rock scarcely needed. His father's "blood enemy" and close friend W. F. "Pooch" Donovan, who had managed the Natick baseball team, the arch rival of Frank Rock's nine, had become coach and trainer at Harvard College. Donovan made Rock promise to go out for some athletic event. Rock complied and won his Harvard letter three times, in his freshman, sophomore, and junior years, in track.

At Harvard, Rock found his Commerce High School courses had prepared him well. In a pinch, he was able to revise some of his high school theme papers, quite acceptably, including the one that won him his South American trip and, interestingly, another on the plight of the American Negro in the work force. Still an ardent Catholic, he attended mass less than daily, but gave substantial time and energy to rejuvenating Harvard's nearly defunct Newman Club, a Catholic students' organization. In his second and third years, he also was a member of Hasty Pudding, Harvard's theatrical society. He performed in two of the society's famous self-styled farces and in two dramas presented in one of Boston's legitimate theaters. He also became a martini maven.

Completing his undergraduate work in three years (to try to catch up for lost time) he graduated with the Harvard class of 1915. Among his classmates were Christian Herter, who twice became governor of Massachusetts and served as secretary of state under Eisenhower. Of more significance for Rock, however, would be Herter's personal championing of his cause nearly fifty years later when Rock took up the cudgel to fight legal and religious disputes over birth control.

Although Rock's scholastic grades at the college were only average, he had no trouble being accepted at Harvard Medical School. In choosing Harvard College as his alma mater, Rock had already become a member of the most important "club" of his life. His loyalty to Harvard would equal that to his Church thenceforward, though neither Harvard nor his Church would return that loyalty to him in such unmeasured terms.

Rock's graduation from medical school in 1918 (his class dubbed themselves the June Brides, an affectionate appellation that followed them throughout their careers) doubly pleased his father. Frank Rock had originally promised his own mother he would try to go to medical school and, further, had promised John's mother he would try to persuade John to do so. As he had with undergraduate school, John Rock completed his formal medical education in three years. The course of study had been accelerated because of World War I.

Along with many of his classmates, Rock was eager to get into the war. He went through extensive examinations for officers training school and was all but accepted. The last hurdle was a recommendation he had to obtain from the medical school. "After long questioning," Rock recalled, "I was standing at the door of the examining professor's office, ready to leave. Everything was approved when he asked, almost as an afterthought, what I would have done had I not gotten my commission. I told him I had an appointment for residency training in surgery at Massachusetts General Hospital. He called me back and took back the approval papers. 'You're not going into the service,' he said. 'Go back to MGH and learn something first.' And so I did."

Following that residency, Rock went on to internships and residencies in obstetrics at Harvard's teaching hospital for maternity medicine, the Boston Lying-In, and for gynecology at the Free Hospital for Women. "There were two fields of medicine that interested me," Rock explained, "the two major functions of humans — cerebration and reproduction. Since cerebration ranks a little higher than reproduction, my first choice was to be a psychiatrist. Then, I acquired a modicum of sense. To become a psychiatrist would have required eight further years of education, study in Europe and all that. Reproduction won out."

Psychiatry, however, remained a strong avocational interest, as did neurology and medical anthropology. Rock, during his college and medical school years, avidly followed the developments coming out of Sigmund Freud's camp in Vienna. He not only admired Freud's thinking but also his daring, particularly his forthright detail concerning the analytic techniques of psychoanalysis. In a 1915 paper entitled "Observations on Transference-Love," Freud wrote — and Rock duly noted — that "Sexual love is undoubtedly one of the chief things in life, and the union of mental and bodily satisfaction in the enjoyment of love is one of its culminating peaks. Apart from a few queer fanatics, all the world knows this and conducts its life accordingly; science alone is too delicate to admit it."

Now, the focus of Rock's life began to crystallize, not only medically, but socially and ethically. It was the duty of the young residents on the obstetrical service to deliver at home the poor pregnant women of the city who came to the Lying-In for their maternity care. For the first time he saw the mean destitution of their lives and the burden imposed by the birth of another unwanted baby they could ill afford to raise. Later, at the Free Hospital for Women, he would see the aftermath of their multiple pregnancies: women with their wombs prolapsing, their kidneys malfunctioning, their bodies misshapen and prematurely old.

One incident above all others remained with him throughout life. He was called to attend a young woman student at Katherine Gibbs secretarial school. She was stricken in her dormitory room, hemorrhaging uncontrollably. "There between her legs was a small, wizened fetus," Rock recalled. "She was terrified. She'd had no idea she was pregnant, nor even knew how a woman became pregnant. I was struck by her ignorance, no, her innocence. I'd had no idea that people knew so little about their own sexuality."

Yet, he had known little himself until his college years. Certainly no one in his family ever told him the facts of life. He was not sure, but assumed he just picked up the information from peers and from books. His own sexual awakening had come fairly late. He remembers the first time he had a spontaneous erection, while working on some audit books for Stone & Webster in their dreary Woonsocket offices. He had to go to the men's room, repeatedly.

During high school he had gradually become aware of "something" that had to be suppressed as sinful, and of course, it was to be confessed. "It was quite a burden to me and I knew it was wrong, but it was uncontrollable. Of course, we had to confess each occasion it happened. I remember picking up that "how to go to confession" book and I began to write down the dates and number of times it occurred, so as to be sure to remember. Finally a priest said to me in the confessional, 'Don't be so scrupulous, John.' "

The priest could not have known Rock very well. He had to be scrupulous. He had known no other way since he was fourteen years old and an encounter took place that shaped the course of his life from that moment on. The event not only touched the deepest corner of his soul, it was to remain there to be called forth whenever he doubted his own scruples, no matter what the issue in question. Years later, he wrote of it:

> In March of 1904 I reach the age of fourteen, so on a Sunday morning I was proudly wearing my first pair of long pants. As I walked out of church after the nine o'clock Mass, Father Finnick, a curate of my parish in Marlborough, Massachusetts, beckoned to me. Very shortly he was to drive to the Poor Farm to make his regular visit. Would I like to go with him? He had taught both our First Communion and our Confirmation class. He was a saintly man, simple and quiet, but a good teacher. Although I had never had anything to do with him outside of class and the confessional, I liked him. . . .
>
> I shall never forget the short slow ride in the small buggy down East Main Street to the Sudbury road, near the beginning of which was the small white building of the Marlborough Poor Farm, were a few very elderly men and women lived.
>
> I don't remember how the conversation started, if you could even call it that. We did not interrupt Father in class, as he gently but firmly expounded Catholic doctrine to us; now, also, I listened intently. I

noticed, as we jogged along, the big Walcott house set back behind a wide lawn. . . .

It was just then he said, "John, always stick to your conscience. Never let anyone else keep it for you." And, after but a moment's pause, he added, "And I mean *anyone* else."

He did not tell me more of it. I guess he knew that I had been in-doctrinated with awareness of the voice of conscience within me, as all Catholics have. He told me to "keep" it.

Rock did just that, as perhaps many men do, but few are called upon to do it so rigorously and at such incredible risk. But in the early 1920s the test of his honor was still far off.

Immediately ahead were more blissful times. Rock had finished preparing for life. Now he was about to undertake living it.

2

FAMILY JOY AND TRAGEDY

ROCK lived exactly according to the tenets he prescribed for everyone else. He had no reason not to; the formula for love, marriage, and parenthood that he proposed to the world had worked for him. Marriage embodied the greatest happiness he would know in life. The children were blue chip dividends. Their home life together was fulfilling beyond his wildest hopes for two unmarred decades.

Anna Thorndike and Rock were introduced by her brother William Sherman (Shermie) Thorndike. He and Rock had become friends as Harvard medical students. Rock knew the first moment he saw her that she was the only one for him. She felt the same instantaneous attraction. They had a magnetism about them that was obvious to everyone, and the spark that ignited between them in that first moment never dimmed.

Her family was a rarity in Boston society. They were Catholic Brahmins, by birth. Her father, Paul Thorndike, was born into the branch of the Thorndike line that had gone west to Milwaukee after the Civil War and later settled in Chicago. They were staunch Protestants, German Lutherans. But her mother, Rachel Sherman — Tecumseh's daughter — was Catholic and the Thorndike children were raised in her faith, as both her church and conscience dictated. When Rock and Nan, as he called her, met, her father, Paul, was Chief of Urology and chief of the service at Boston City Hospital.

Even though she grew up in an *Upstairs, Downstairs* style household of white gloves and engraved calling cards deposited on silver trays in the hallway, Anna Thorndike was not typical of the young women of her day. She insisted upon substance in her life. After graduating from a finishing school, she demanded a genuine education and majored in mathematics at Bryn Mawr. She was very unlike her sister Martha, who was named debutante of the year and relished that sort of social distinction and all that went with it. Anna, however, was more like her mother, who though undeniably a positioned member of Boston's socialite set, exerted her own independence in her own way. Rachel Sherman Thorndike, for example, was among the first to "take in" the New Yorker Isabella Stewart Gardner, who, at first, was snubbed unmercifully by Boston socialites after her marriage to multimillionaire Jack Gardner. Not only did Isabella and Rachel become close friends, they indulged in outrageous pastimes for socialite women, often smoking cigars or pipes of tobacco in public.

Before marrying Rock, Anna Thorndike exhibited much of the same adventurous spirit her husband-to-be had shown in his early sojourns in Central and South America. She went off to France during World War I as an ambulance driver at the age of twenty, in 1916. Not only was she an expert driver long before most women even thought of driving a car, she could take a car motor apart and put it back together again. In 1923 she returned to France as a member of the Comité Americain pour les Régions Dévastées de la France. For her service overseas she was awarded the French government's Médaille de la Reconnaissance. Her overseas duty led to a special bond of friendship with Rock's twin sister, Nell, who, also, had been a Red Cross driver during the war years.

John and Nan had to abide a frustratingly long courtship, though it had its sweet moments. "We often would visit at Harvard [Massachusetts] where her family had a summer place. I loved to dance, but Nan didn't take to it too well. Just the same, she'd go to the assemblies with me and we had a great time together with Shermie and Martha and my sister Nell and her husband, Charlie Mulloy." It was a long wait for young medical school graduates in those days before they could entertain thoughts of marriage for they received no pay for their internships or residency training periods. To get money to live on, immediately after graduation Rock signed on as an assistant to a general surgeon, Dr. Sam Goddard, in the shoe-factory city of Brockton. One of life's coincidences at the time brought him into contact with Hudson Hoagland, the neurobiologist, who later would co-found with Gregory Pincus the Worcester Foundation for Experimental Biology. By chance, Rock was called to administer the anesthesia, while Dr. Ray Titus of Boston attended the birth of Hoagland's first son, Mahlon. (Later, it was to be through Hoagland, that the mission to find a contraceptive pill would bring Rock and Pincus into collaboration.) By the time Rock finished his multiple residencies in general surgery, urology, obstetrics, and gynecology, he felt so old that he "thought it was time to start practice and support myself. Besides, I was yearning to marry Nan."

He was appointed an assistant in Obstetrics at Harvard Medical School in 1922. The next year, encouraged by MGH colleagues, he reactivated the MGH's infertility clinic, a reflection of where his research interest already was leading. In 1924, he started a new infertility clinic at the Free Hospital for Women, where he had received a staff appointment and where he would make highly significant original contributions to new knowledge about human reproduction. It was at this point, with a private obstetrical and gynecological practice developing, that he finally could afford to marry his dear "great, gawky girl."

When they were planning their wedding, her father suggested they go to see his old friend from medical school days, a young priest, who as a curate in St. Joseph's parish in the North End had lived in the same boardinghouse that Paul Thorndike had lived in while a young medical resident. The priest had become William Cardinal O'Connell. The cardinal asked them where they were planning to be married. "We mentioned St. Cecilia's in the Back Bay," Rock fondly remembered. "And the cardinal said, 'No, it shall be at Immaculate Conception [a magnificent Boston cathedral] and I shall marry you.'" He did, on January 3, 1925, in one of the most publicized weddings of the decade. Streets were roped off for blocks around because the cardinal did not customarily perform marriage ceremonies. The only couple whom he had so honored up to that time had been Joseph and Rose Kennedy.

Though only the immediate members of the family knew it, Rock went through a minor crisis in faith the day before the elaborate wedding. He'd been performing cesarean sections, delivery of babies through a surgical incision rather than vaginally, a practice then forbidden by the Church. (One of the reasons the Church frowned on cesarean sections at the turn of the century was because they had become fashionable among well-to-do European women who did not want to undergo the pain of childbirth. To bear children in pain was, of course, womankind's inheritance, the price of Eve's fall from grace in Eden. Not until Queen Victoria accepted chloroform during her confinements was the practice given Protestant sanction, either.) At confession, the priest refused to give Rock absolution. Unless he straightened the matter out, technically he could not receive the sacrament of marriage the following day. There was great consternation in the family. At the wedding rehearsal, his soon to be mother-in-law, Rachel Thorndike, mentioned it to Cardinal O'Connell, who guffawed and immediately conferred absolution. Instead of calming Rock down, however, the act disturbed him. In those days, such casualness over a sinful matter was enough to disconcert a Catholic. Supposedly, rules of behavior were not to be changeable from priest to priest.

As young newlyweds, Rock and his bride lived temporarily in apartments in Brookline and in Boston's Back Bay. Rock was already thirty-five and his wife, twenty-nine, when they wed, and they started the family they both wanted the very first year. It was at their Massachusetts Avenue Back Bay apartment that Rock's colleagues at the Free Hospital for Women and his lifetime friends Drs. George and Olive Smith first visited them. Over the years, the Rocks' and the Smiths' lives were interwoven, both professionally and personally, though they were not always to agree, scientifically. Within another year, Rock was to buy the family home, a home he could not really afford. Money considerations, however, seldom influenced anything he wanted to do.

The Rock house was a big comfortable place, set well back off the road on Quail Street in West Roxbury. The property had been part of the vast estate originally owned by the Codman brothers, scions of a prominent Boston family of financiers. It was bordered on one side by the woods and flowerlands of the several-hundred-acre Arnold Arboretum, Harvard's renowned botanical gardens, and extended on the other side over rolling lawns down to the main road into Boston. Rock bought one of the Codman houses and Roxbury Latin School (the oldest private school in America) bought the other two.

Done in the manner of a French country manor, the double-winged Rock house was stucco, outlined in heavy, dark-stained wood. There were six rooms downstairs, seven bedrooms up and five baths. The entrance hallway was a room in itself, plus a large dining room and a thirty-foot living room, "so tremendous," his daughters recall, that they could and did ride their first bicycles around in it. The family laundry was hung to dry (as Mrs. Lincoln did in the White House) in a cavernous attic.

The five Rock children were born in fairly rapid succession. Rachel Sherman Rock was the first, born on December 30, 1925, just eleven months after her parents were wed. John Jr. came next, born July 15, 1927. Eighteen months later, Ann Jane arrived on January 7, 1929. Martha followed within sixteen months on May 4, 1930, and Ellen, the youngest, less than three years later on February 21, 1933.

"The house was always full of dogs (mostly boxers) and children," is the way George and Olive Smith remembered it. "They had these five children quite quickly and they were devils, complete!" One evening when the Smiths were dining with the Rocks, the children "got on the loose and painted the bathroom with India ink. John thought that was very funny. There wasn't much that could get him angry." The Smiths, a husband-wife research team at the Free Hospital, were of a totally different temperament. They did not see quite the same "felicitous humor" in the Rock children's behavior that John and Nan did.

For their generation, Rock and his wife were exceptional parents as well as exceptional individuals in their own right. They permitted their children great freedom, as their own parents had allowed them: a freedom based on utter confidence in the childrens' own worth. The parental philosophy held that the children were all intelligent and therefore, once they were taught and understood right from wrong, surely they would do what was right and become good and honorable people. The rest was just good, healthy self-expression, which never failed to delight their doting parents.

The children were fortunate and they knew it. They lived within walking distance of stores, libraries, and movie theaters; Boston's concert halls, museums, and special events were only a trolley ride away. Yet, their house and yard was entered along a long, private unpaved dirt lane, edged by a woodland more customarily found in the countryside. It was ideal. Along with dogs, the children had practically every other kind of pet, including ducks, which were always getting loose and running off. The children also raised rabbits. On another of the Smiths' dinner visits, George recalled, "we dined on some of the rabbits. The meal was delicious, but this bothered us because of our years of using rabbits in our research." The Rocks may well have been putting the Smiths on by serving them rabbit. It was the kind of family joke they would have conspired to play with great gusto.

As parents, John and Nan Rock presided over their family like the reigning heads of a benevolent kingdom. As a pair they were marvelously suited to one another. Even physically and temperamentally, they were much alike. "Mother was six feet tall; Daddy, six one and a half. Both were extremely intelligent. She weighed around one hundred eighty pounds without being fat in any way. That was her normal size. She was very beautiful. Not in a *Playboy* magazine sense, of course, but as a big, strong, handsome woman with a big strong face," daughter Ann Jane, or AJ as she is known, recalled. "The two of them were so good looking, with truly commanding presence, posture, poise, dash. . . . Even their voices were commanding. Those two walking into a room at a party or on some special occasion would stop the room cold!"

As a couple they loved each other deeply and exclusively. They epitomized the meaning of monogamy. Their devotion to one another had nothing to do with duty or obligation; they adored being together. He thought her utterly remarkable, "superior in every way." She returned this view of him.

He was an enlightened husband at a time when most men regarded their wive's lot in life as being content with bearing and rearing children and doing housework. Not Rock. He was sensitive to the burdens of motherhood his wife bore and to the rigors of running their household. He also recognized her need to be herself and use the fine mind she possessed. "I always wanted her to go back and teach math at a university. She was a mathematical genius. Instead, she married me and became a champion bridge player. She taught me to play or tried to. She said I had card sense. But I wasn't really interested — except in her and to be with her."

Rock was an unmitigated romantic. He relished the byplay that goes on — or should — between men and women in love. He delighted in selecting just the right flowers: a perfect lily, a magenta azalea, a bowl of burnt orange nasturtiums. He always celebrated anniversaries of every sort with choice personal remembrances. He never passed up the quick, stolen hug in the hallway when guests were in the living room. He particularly savored sharing the day's goings-on over a chilled, silver shaker of martinis, which he and Nan partook of during the "quiet hour" they reserved for one another each and every evening they were together throughout their married life.

Money was never plentiful, even though to outsiders it seemed the Rocks lived as if it were. There was no "old money" inheritance, although there should have been. The family story goes that old Tecumseh Sherman entrusted his estate to an elderly bachelor brother for safekeeping. The brother, however, surprisingly married late in life and left it all to his relatively new wife, cutting out Tecumseh's daughter Rachel and her Thorndike progeny. Rock's father, in turn, had gone through all the family real estate holdings in Marlborough during the Depression years, using up the last of it in Florida where he had retired with Delia and eventually died. Rock's financially successful brother Charlie even had to forward train tickets so that John could travel to their father's deathbed.

All that John Rock's family had to live on were his earnings. Though he could have made a small fortune with his practice in which he became the foremost expert in his field of infertility, he paid little to no attention to bill collecting. As a student, he had become accustomed to patients' not paying for their care, and he never got out of the frame of mind that it was a doctor's duty to provide free care. A good doctor should neither want nor expect to make money on other people's unfortunate illnesses, he believed. Once, one of his secretaries helped herself to the patients' payments, pocketing the cash amounts for herself for months. Rock never noticed until he underwent a routine audit for the hospital's purposes. Then, he was stuck with paying back quite a lot more in back taxes on the misappropriated income. Rather than being furious, Rock was characteristically "just disappointed." He could see how the secretary was tempted and refused to press charges. Thereafter, however, he changed the bookkeeping system.

During the 1930s, when the children were young, Rock's practice was starting to build, but the country meantime was strapped by the Great Depression, and many patients, including many of Rock's, simply could not pay their doctor's bills. But Mrs. Rock managed to provide the family with healthy seaside vacations by working as the manager of the Nahant Inn for three years. Later, she taught bridge to classes of twenty and thirty people during weekday afternoons at the Quail Street house. Nothing was beneath her. Although accustomed to servants as a Thorndike daughter, she pitched in wherever needed as Rock's wife. She ran the house with help when they could afford it and alone when they couldn't. "She did important things like paint storm windows, scrape and refinish furniture, and paint walls," Rock recalled. "But it never bothered her. It truly never did." The family often was financially strapped however, as the Great Depression took hold. She was the manager. After John went off to the hospital around six in the morning, stopping for mass and communion on the way, she distributed the children at their various schools. Rock, in his formally descriptive way, referred to it as "a certain substratum of conventionality. It all ran very, very smoothly."

During the economically stressful early years, and later when finances improved, Rock and his wife always made time not only for family and work, but also for social self-fulfillment. Mrs. Rock played bridge in masters' tournaments, was a long-time member of the Boston Committee of the Frontier Nursing Service. (In the 1960s Rock interceded with the Searle Company to provide the frontier nurses in Appalachia and Kentucky with free supplies of the pill.) She also was active in the Bryn Mawr Club of Boston and the Social Service Committee of Boston City Hospital, Boston's medically famed municipal hospital for the poor. During World War II, she was a Red Cross canteen volunteer in Boston, serving on the docks passing out doughnuts and coffee to servicemen on their way overseas. Rock belonged to the Harvard Club as a matter of form, and also was an ardent member of the Tavern Club in Boston, a private men's club of great distinction. Tucked almost out of view at the far end of a blind alleyway called Boylston Place, the Tavern Club catered to the wealthy and well-positioned. Few Catholics were invited to join, but Rock says his father-in-law Paul Thorndike got both him and "Shermie" Thorndike in in 1927, when "the membership was getting superannuated and they needed some new young blood." It was Rock's favorite milieu. He took great delight in the casual manner in which members were required to sit down for lunch at the first table they encountered. Everyone was on a first-name basis.

The Tavern Club also afforded a private and protected outlet for him to express his avocational theatrical talents over the years. He took part in most of the Tavern's three annual productions, many of them musicals and all written and produced by members. "He was the bane and the hit of every show, learning his lines only cursorily, and then improving on them as he improvised along the way," according to Dr. Curtis Prout, dean of students at Harvard Medical School, and a lifelong Taverner. "His version was always funnier, but it raised hell with the cues." Rock rarely missed the weekly Monday night dinner meeting, and frequently stopped by for lunch. "He always lit up the room, the second he arrived," said Monsignor Francis J. Lally, former editor of the Boston *Pilot,* the archdiocesan newspaper, and presently Secretary of the Department of Social Development and World Peace for the U.S. Catholic Conference in Washington, D.C. Rock proposed Tavern membership for Lally, the first priest ever accepted.

From 1949 on when he was voted in to the even more exclusive Medical Exchange Club founded in 1920, he also made time for its once-a-month meetings. For years, membership was limited to no more than twelve members, each preeminent in his medical specialty. Among the select few, were three Boston Nobelists. The existence of the club was not well known, even to Boston's close-knit medical community. The members met customarily in one another's homes, each meeting the occasion for a sumptuous gourmet dinner, replete with the best liquors, wines, and cordials; members took turns giving informal reports on their front-line research or some cultural topic. More than mere colleagues, members were best friends. They were frankly snobbish, occasionally revealing their stereotyped social prejudices, and they could be insufferably precious about some of their personal pursuits. But they all were important in medicine's big league.

While Rock was a part of the medical aristocracy of the time, he was about to "break form" by standing out alone on a delicate issue of the times: the fight which was about to begin over birth control. In the sexually permissive climate of today, it is almost impossible to appreciate the emotional, moral, political and religious fervor that the subject of birth control aroused at that time. While a ban on birth control is now most strongly associated with Roman Catholicism and fundamentalist Protestant and Muslim sects, few are aware that the same prohibition was imposed by nearly all Protestant denominations, though perhaps less menacingly, until 1930.

During the first quarter of the century, however, a new and vibrant humanism was beginning to stir in the Western world, a more liberal attitude born of fresh insights into human sexuality emanating from the discoveries of Sigmund Freud and his followers in the new field of psychology; from the equally new sciences of sociology and economics; and from the rebirth of Malthusian thought with its grim vision of a world outgrowing its food supply and overpopulating itself into mass starvation.

Onto the world stage also marched Margaret Sanger, the single most ardent and relentless causist for family planning and a one-woman force to be reckoned with. In 1913 she founded the Birth Control League (later to become the International Planned Parenthood Federation) to fight openly for legalized contraception, particularly for impoverished women entrapped by the industrialized revolution and the tenement life it spawned.

The turning point in condemnation of birth control as an un-

Christian act came at the Lambeth Conference of 1930. That name was given the world assembly of bishops of the Anglican Church held once every decade at Lambeth Palace, the official residence of the Archbishop of Canterbury. While the conference does not promulgate official doctrine, as does the Papacy for Catholics, its pronouncements on matters of faith and morals constitute the consensus of the higher Anglican clergy.

There, for the first time, the changing opinions of the times concerning the morality of birth control prevailed among any body of Christian clergy. Despite hardline opposition, the conference on August 15 adopted by a significant majority a resolution that favored a limited acceptance of contraception.

The reasons and conditions set by the conference which were to govern the practice of contraception remained very strict, and were amazingly close to latter-day thinking of the Roman Catholic Church. The central section of the historic Lambeth resolution said:

> Where there is a clearly felt moral obligation to limit or avoid parenthood the method must be decided on Christian principles. The primary and obvious method is complete abstinence from intercourse (as far as may be necessary) in a life of discipline and self-control lived in the power of the Holy Spirit. Nevertheless in those cases where there is such a clearly-felt moral obligation to limit or avoid parenthood, and where there is morally sound reason for avoiding complete abstinence, the Conference agrees that other methods may be used, provided this is done in the light of the same Christian principles. The Conference records its strong condemnation of conception control from motives of selfishness, luxury or mere convenience.

The time span for similar acceptance of contraception by other Protestant sects stretched out over another three decades, until 1959 when the practice was finally approved by the World Council of Churches.

One undenied effect of the 1930 Lambeth Conference revision of its stance on contraception was to prod the Roman Catholic leadership of that day into promulgating its first definitive statement on birth control. It came in the form of the papal encyclical, *Casti Canubii,* issued by Pope Pius XI on the last day of the year, December 31, 1930. Although it was not pronounced *ex cathedra,* and thus did not carry the totally binding weight of papal infallibility, nonetheless it would be the operative rule for the half billion Roman Catholics across the world.

In a word, Pius XI said no to birth control by any "artificial" means for Catholics, and further, affirmed that it was intrinsically wrong, for anyone, as murder is. He discounted any justification for the practice: "Assuredly no reason, even the most serious, can make congruent with nature and decent what is intrinsically against nature."

One offshoot of the Protestant approval of birth control, a gain immediately seized upon by the birth control crusader Margaret Sanger and her Birth Control League, was a petition in 1931 to repeal Massachusetts's anti–birth control law. Opposition to any repeal of the ban was just as forcefully mustered in response to the consequent 1930 papal encyclical *Casti Canubii*.

Rock was a unique figure in the drama. He was the only Catholic among fifteen of Boston's leading physicians who signed the petition. In six years, he had come a long way, philosophically, from the day before his wedding when he anguished over the personal sin of having performed a cesarean section. Two advances in medical thinking had altered his own — permanently.

Until the 1920s, birth control came down basically to the ancient maneuver, premature withdrawal, or condoms, which had come in with the vulcanization of rubber in 1843, or the "modern" method, the diaphragm, developed in 1880. But in the mid-1920s, a new concept in contraception — timing — was added to the standard armamentarium. Independent of one another, two scientists — Kyasaku Ogino in Japan in 1924 and Herman Knaus in Austria in 1927 — had learned that a woman's fertile period occurred approximately midway in her monthly menstrual cycle. For a woman with a regular menstrual cycle, it became possible to avoid intercourse selectively, when conception might occur. The new information formed the basis of "rhythm," the avoidance of pregnancy by abstaining from sex relations during the fertile period. An entirely new moral question now had to be confronted. Since intercourse could morally be enjoyed during pregnancy, or after menopause — times when conception could not occur — would the same reasoning apply to sterile periods during the menstrual cycle? Without specifically referring to rhythm, Pope Pius XI had noted in the 1930 encyclical that sexual abstinence for short or prolonged periods was permissible when it was necessary to avoid pregnancy for very serious reasons. In Rock's view, the answer was: of course. Were not all the sterile periods natural? Why should taking advantage of one differ from another?

Further, his own research focus into possible avenues to overcome infertility in women so they could conceive and bear children had led him into very serious consideration of the opposite. He became convinced that some women suffered from an equally abnormal opposite state, which he termed overfertility. Oddly no one has followed up his perception of overfertility as a valid reproductive abnormality. In the Yankee-dominated Harvard setting where he practiced, little attention was paid, somewhat understandably, to Catholic couples with that problem. Neither, however, did their own Catholic hospitals. Rock alone acted. In 1936, shortly after the basis for the new "rhythm" method was propounded, he opened the first "rhythm" clinic in the United States, and possibly the world, to teach Catholic women how to calculate the fertile period in their menstrual period so they could try to avoid pregnancy. The method had not been formally approved by the Church and would not be for another twenty years, but he correctly anticipated it would be because it was based both on a natural biologic condition and on sexual abstinence. He knew from firsthand observation the hardships that repeated pregnancy imposed on poor and often sick women, and he acted on his belief that "Nature never intended a woman to be pregnant over and over again."

He not only had signed the 1931 petition to do away with the state's birth control ban, he did so openly and was outspoken in support of legalizing birth control and of placing the decision in the hands of the woman and her doctor. In so doing, he aligned himself with the Planned Parenthood "crowd," a despicable group in Catholic eyes. His stance within the Boston archdiocese was worse than sinful, it was traitorous! The Catholic community couldn't comprehend that he was trying to make "rhythm" work for Catholics, since all other forms of "artificial" birth control — condoms, diaphragms, foams, jellies, and even coitus interruptus — were forbidden them and he did not accept the rightness of imposing Catholic birth control restrictions on non-Catholics. But Rock had no trouble with his conscience over the birth control petition. "I separated biology from theology quite early in my life," he said of the episode later, "and never confused them again."

AJ's first realization that her father was an "important" man came from her first brush with the animosity he generated among some local clergy. One summer day AJ and her brother, Jack, were hitchhiking from home in West Roxbury to the Longwood Cricket Club in Chestnut Hill, Brookline, which the Rocks had joined to make sure the children had a place to swim for the summer. A priest picked them up to give them a lift home. "Jack was eleven or so and I was just ten," AJ recalled. "As we were riding along, the priest asked our name. When learned who we were, he told us we'd have to get out. He said, 'I cannot have the children of John Rock in my car.' " Their attitude was, "Too bad for you. If Daddy didn't care what people said about him, neither did we."

The Rocks went to extreme lengths to make sure their children were as intellectually educated in Catholicism as they were in secular subjects. On the one occasion when their youngest daughter, Ellen, returned from Sunday school at their parish, St. Theresa's, they were horrified. As she told her parents what the lesson was, they realized she was being woefully misinstructed. "The gist of the lesson," Ellen vividly remembered, "was that only Catholics would go to Heaven. Well, that's sheer heresy. The Roman Catholic Church has never taught that and you can be sure my father and mother were not going to have any of their children exposed to such nonsense. That was the first and last day for me at that Sunday school."

That Ellen was sent to the local parish for religious instruction merely reflected Mrs. Rock's weariness. For years, she had driven the older children weekly to the Cenacle Retreat House, a Catholic discussion center in Newton. Only World War II with its gasoline and tire shortages ended the weekly trips. Thereafter, Mrs. Rock hired a lay Catholic teacher to come to the Rock house weekly to tutor the children in Catholicism. "When I had questions she couldn't answer," AJ says, "Mrs. Ellis would make an appointment for me with a Jesuit professor of philosophy at Boston College." Prior to that, "Mom drove a half an hour each way every Sunday from West Roxbury to Newton and then sat in the back of the car reading a book so that we would have the best teaching in our religion. To do that for five children? My God!"

It was no different for the Rock children's secular education. Mrs. Rock investigated the schools, then she and Rock discussed the options and picked the best that could be found — and afforded. In a big old station wagon, every morning, Mrs. Rock, sometimes still in her nightgown and wrapper, would drive the children to their various schools. At the end of the day, she'd retrieve them, often chauffeuring them to other activities along the way. Partly because of its educational excellence and partly because of the wartime gasoline and tire shortages, by the 1940s all of the Rock children went to one school, Milton Academy. That way one trip took care of them all. All boys were eligible to board there, so Jack did. (Girls had to live more than fifty miles away.) The tuition was only a fraction of costs today, "but," as Rachel points out, "it was still pretty heavy stuff financially, with five of us to carry."

It was in the midst of this tuition load that Rock suffered a near fatal heart attack. His coronary drove home the perilous financial state of the household, the awareness of which became the linchpin of Rock's recovery. If he died, his family would be left in dire straits. There were no pensions, no annuities, no disability provisions for Harvard academics and their families in those days. The heart attack struck in May 1944 and Rock wasn't released from the Phillips House at MGH until the following September. He was fifty-four. The coronary was the first of six he would endure and survive.

As with other challenges he confronted he weighed the situation and adjusted it to his own sense of what would work. The standard treatment for heart attack victims in that era was prolonged bed rest. He didn't have time to be away from his practice and earning money for the family. He stayed a shorter and again a shorter time in the hospital after the second and third heart attacks, signing himself out when he deemed himself ready. After that, when he was stricken less severely, he and Nan simply went up to the Groton Inn in the restful countryside near Groton School and "took it easy" for a few weeks.

Because heart attack victims were forbidden any strenuous exercise, he figured out a way to get exercise passively. Daily, he'd have Nan drive him a few miles to "Drop-Kick" Murphy's "dry-out farm" for alcoholics, named for its ex-football star owner, and have vigorous body massages. They not only were therapeutic, but also relaxing and enjoyable. Why not? Turning adversity into advantage was his way. From then on, wherever he was on his travels or at home, he had body massages "to exercise his arteries, you understand," every chance he got.

When he returned to his practice, he gave up obstetrics. He could no longer tax himself with being called out at any hour of the day or night to deliver babies. His nitroglycerin tablets to stave off heart attacks became his lifeline. And he took them with greater frequency than was probably needed, popping them beneath his tongue at the slightest provocation. One of his research associates, Dr. Herbert "Trader" Horne, recalled a day when "Rock came to the office and just sat perfectly immobile in his chair. In a barely audible voice so as not to strain himself in the slightest way, he told me he'd forgotten his bottle of nitroglycerin. He wouldn't move, not an inch, until I raced across the street to the hospital and fetched him a new supply. As soon as I handed them to him, he bounced right up and got going, the moment he knew they were at hand's reach."

It seems strange, but his family was not overly concerned that he would push himself into another heart attack. "He didn't work that way," according to his daughter Rachel, who worked at the Free Hospital for Women at the time. "He didn't push. He worked terribly hard, but he was a master at pacing himself. I don't remember that he ever overdid. He just budgeted his time with infinite care. He ate lunch at his desk, dictated notes between patients, checked over research results before he came home each night." His appointment books show that he sometimes rationed his time slots for phone calls and letters down to five-minute segments. He maximized whatever time was available. After the 1944 heart attack, he also reversed his operating-room schedule, making hospital rounds first at 7:30 A.M., because still sleepy patients took up less of his time in idle conversation that way. He always had a dozen projects working simultaneously, and he juggled them all very deftly.

But life has a way of catching up with everyone and the Rocks were no exception. The halcyon years of the 1930s left them unprepared for the brutal shock to come. Rock was still recovering from his heart attack when it happened. His only son, John Jr., or Jack as he was called by the family, a lance-corporal in the U.S. Marine Corps, died in an automobile accident. It happened the day before he was to be discharged from the service.

On Sunday, August 13, 1946, he had come home on a pass and had dinner with his parents. Even though the evening was growing late, his father urged him to go on to a party for disabled servicemen, which was being held in Sherbourne, some twenty miles away. Rachel had gone earlier to the party at the home of friends of the Rocks. Rock remembers that Rachel called to ask him to send Jack along to help entertain by playing the piano. Jack was dog tired, but gave in to his father's urging to go give his sister a hand.

It was late when he arrived at the party, but he quickly met everyone. The servicemen all were patients at the Cushing General Army Hospital in Framingham. He played the piano for them as long as they wanted him to. "He really wasn't there very long," Rachel recalls, "but when we left in separate cars, we both were going to drop people off at their homes. Some of them lived quite a distance away." It was a nasty night, pitch dark and pouring rain.

Jack's last stop was way out in Millis where he dropped a girl off at her house. He headed back for Portsmouth, where he was due back on duty at 6 A.M. "He was driving alone along terribly wet, dark, winding roads. He missed a curve and crashed headlong into a tree," his sister recalled. He suffered a severe head injury and developed a fever of 107 degrees. Dr. Donald Munro, the Harvard professor and MGH neurosurgeon, was called as a consultant and he was "not encouraging." Jack's temperature continued to climb, uncontrollably. "Even if he had lived," Rachel acknowledges calmly now, "he would surely have been a vegetable. He died that Tuesday night, August fifteenth, just a month to the day after his nineteenth birthday."

Rock never recovered from the heartbreak — or self-imposed guilt — of that loss. He blamed himself. "It was really my fault, you know. Jack said he was very tired, but I encouraged him to go, saying his sister was counting on him. I don't break down anymore if I concentrate on it," he said pointing to a smiling photograph of the young man hanging on the bedroom wall facing his bed. "I can look at the picture, finally. He was a great kid."

By the time of Rock's fiftieth class reunion in 1965, he could note that he had taken the advice he so often gave his bereaved childless patients, to look to "other sources of happiness." He chose the language of theatrical troupers: "But the show had to go on. After two dreadful years, I acquired in 1948, the first of four splendid sons-in-law. My recovery from the deadening loss of my son had taught me that life might still be worth living. I didn't quite believe it. It has turned out to be partly true."

Only their own sense of themselves, their invincible faith, and their own resistance over the years to what the outside world thought of them saw the Rock family through their terrible loss. Down deep, they had grit and they expressed their sorrow at home in private and kept going. Beyond their own circle, they behaved the same as always — good-humored, pleasantly urbane, and unruffled.

Rock's heartbreak over the death of his son, so close and dear to him and so young, could not but have enhanced his concern for family life — for the meaning of children — and for the human sexuality that propels them into being. Rock was the most passionate of believers in family life and a supreme advocate of love between man and woman — husband for wife, parents for their children. The real problem was that there were few in society, not to mention religious life, who had the faintest grasp of what Rock well knew love and life were all about.

From long professional experience with couples tormented by being childless or overprolific, he knew the need for their love to be strong and continuously reinforced by sexual union. He drew from his own personal love of spouse, and the physical intimacy that such love fed on, to think through his conclusions on the true nature of human sexuality.

Love of one's mate is the quality, more than any other, that separates man from the lower animals, he became certain. The capacity to love is an expression of Man's intellectual and spiritual evolution. Human love is the essential quality that distinguishes the human sex act from purely instinctive animal sex. "Too many sacerdotes still confuse the incredibly profound meaning of human coitus with what they view as degrading animalistic copulation," he said. Rock knew better. In an essay, "Sex, Science and Survival," prepared as the seventh Oliver Bird Lecture and presented at the London School of Hygiene and Tropical Medicine in 1963, Rock reflected on what he had learned about love and the family: "I have studied, researched and tried to solve problems in Man's pervasive sexuality, the biological requisite for species survival. Common to most animals is some form of sex for propagation. Hence it is that Man is equipped (we cannot in our present dilemma unqualifiedly say 'endowed,' and most of us are not yet willing to say, 'cursed') with a powerful urge to copulate." Rock saw human sexuality as part and parcel of the gynecologist's professional domain. "The gynecologist (rightly) has much to do with Man's copulatory urge."

Rock had never shrunk from the subject of human sexuality in his professional practice, though that idea was anathema to the medical profession in his era, and sex remains a discomfiting and not quite respectable subject for many physicians even now. He, however, had stood virtually alone as one of the early pioneers in the field of human sexual behavior, one that the majority of his colleagues in the 1920s, '30s and '40s considered unsavory, if not downright salacious, for a gentleman, not to mention a physician, to be concerned with. To Rock, however, sex was the bedrock upon which love in marriage was built. With typically openminded curiosity and the courage of his ethical convictions, he became certain that frequent and enjoyable sex was natural, necessary, and above all, the *highest* expression of marital love. Rock peeled away the shrouds of secrecy and unwarranted shame that the society of his day kept the subject of sex embalmed in. He summed up his lifetime observations on the place of sex in the human experience this way: "The basic normal male, stripped of social, experiential and — shall we say — spiritual repressions is as sexually promiscuous and ruminative as any ape; and like the ape, he is only very temporarily satiated. He is physically superior and is ever desirous and potent. For untold centuries moralists have used whatever social pressures they could bring to bear on the human male's coital urge in efforts to restrict its expression outside marriage. Recent news media reflect the degree of their failure," he observed. Then, he pointed out, as only sexologist Kinsey had up to that time (and Masters and Johnson would reconfirm in 1966), his unpopular but correct observation: that the healthy female was equally as strongly compelled by sex as the male. "The problem [of population control] is complicated further by the fact that, basically, the normal woman, if similarly bereft of social, experiential and spiritual inhibitions, although physically weaker, has deep within her an ever-present willingness, and often, like the male — an *urge* to copulate."

Love, he argued, was the transcendent value, the peculiarly human attribute that tempered "the savage, anthropoid core of sexuality in the human being today. In the evolution of the hominid from his apelike progenitors . . . there arose . . . not only the powerful coital urge, but also the utterly particular emotional quality of love." Conceding that few could define love, "the greatest of the three virtues," he acknowledged, "we are all aware, that, in various forms, it characterizes us as human beings. Inseparable from our human sexuality, because it is an integral part of it however obscured, is love: love of mate and love of young." Then, with full assuredness, he stated: "Only when love of mate suffuses coitus does orgasm reach its natural fullness of ecstasy." Thereafter, he went on, "it is the love of young which motivates informed, intelligent, responsible, mutually loving parents to reproduce instead of merely to procreate." Animals could procreate and replace their kind mindlessly. It was for humans to reproduce an elevated human being such as themselves, which bound parents to provide care, protection, and education for each child brought into the world. On a quieter note, he expressed his personal though professionally supported view: "I would suppose that the inherency of love within the human sex instinct is responsible for near universality of monogamy." All the experts — archaeologists, anthropologists, and sociologists — he noted, "report this mating form in practically all races, in all places, and all times."

"It seems quite clear that monogamy is the ideal modal social unit of the human race. Could it be," he asked rhetorically, "that through long ages, intelligent Man learned that monogamous marriage of loving mates offers the best opportunity for perfect expression of the peculiarly human qualities of the sex instinct? In monogamous marriage of loving mates, they can both find full gratification of the two inseparable components of their instinct — the coital urge, and the love that unites them and that impels them healthfully to rear and productively to educate their offspring."

That's the way it was for Rock and for his wife. They carefully and knowingly cultivated their connubial love so that they would be so inextricably bonded together, they would have the strength to bear and raise their children, properly. Rock defined what that meant in the Bird Lecture, too: "Intellectually mature human beings do not reproduce, do not multiply themselves (according to the Biblical injunction) when they merely beget. The job is not done, nor can it be done, until such parents have produced sons and daughters with understanding and free will." In the Rock family household, the emphasis was given equally to those considerations: understanding and free will.

Looking back, Rock's daughters' biggest complaint is that it often seemed to them as children that their father was never home. Six days a week he left before they were up in the morning and did not return before seven in the evening. In his diaries, however, it is clear that he took an enormous interest in the children. When they went to summer camp he wrote them faithfully, long letters filled with devotion, as he did his wife, whenever he was away on lecture trips or scientific meetings. But the great fun came around the dinner table on Sundays and special occasions when guests were present. "Daddy usually held forth and the rest of us listened," Rachel says, "but Daddy was never particularly close-mouthed regarding sex and reproduction." His discussions, though completely within the bounds of good taste, were totally frank. Sometimes their mother had to explain later precisely what some of it meant, however. Without mentioning names, he frequently talked with the family about his work and some of his cases. One of their favorite stories concerned a young couple who had just had a full-sized, full-term pudgy baby boy. The problem was that the baby had been borne after they had only been married seven months. They were terrified that their parents would find out that the baby was conceived out of wedlock. Rock took care of the problem for them. He enlisted the help of the nurses and had the baby transferred to the "preemie" nursery, and made sure it was kept well-wrapped in receiving blankets, so that not much of the baby's round full face showed. He then met the grandparents and took them to see the newborn, assuring them that the baby, though a bit premature, would be just fine. "Why not?" he laughed. "The poor young couple shouldn't have had to have a silly problem like that on their mind to spoil their happiness." It was a grand and innocent canard, just the kind of subterfuge that made him the favorite doctor of all the nurses on the hospital staff.

On the surface it would appear that Rock and his wife's efforts to instill in their children their own unshakable faith in Catholicism failed. Only Ellen remains a practicing Catholic. Rock and his wife were of an older school, whose Catholicism was unmovable despite any "annoying clerics" they might encounter. Nan had been brought up in the French-tradition Catholic Church, which was more liberal than the Irish-American Catholic tradition in which Rock was raised. But Rock in time became impatient with what he saw as the petty-minded thinking of many priests, who, he said, submitted to "the urge to escape as many of the handicaps [of life] as possible by withdrawing from the world, from all worldliness, from all society, as have many of every known religion. It is easy [for them] to think in the abstract . . . of what was right and what was wrong in how a person willed, or permitted, or prevented the expression of his God-given sexuality. I suggest it is not easy for any descendent of Adam to achieve this complete submission."

Yet, in a deeper sense, the lessons of the parents took, but are expressed by their daughters with characteristic family individuality. Each daughter knows a deep spirituality, ethical responsibility, and intensely humane personal philosophy. What Rock's daughters have done is take their early Catholic training beyond the narrow confines of traditional expression. That ultimately is what their parents wanted — for them to find their own sense of religion. Their daughters say they just have been less willing than their parents to put up with the mediocrity of small-minded clerics. On the large issues, Rock's daughters indeed did keep faith with their parents' religious and social convictions. They are honest to a fault. They, too, have mated once and for always. They raise their children with freedom and zest for life and that special brand of courtesy, true concern for others, that Rock exemplified.

"One of the things about Daddy is that he was a totally human man. Nor as a doctor did he forget that people are humans. He did not just try to solve their medical problems, he tried to help them to be happy.

He knew that they couldn't have a good married life when they had unsatisfactory sex relations," Ellie once said. "In those days many people didn't know anything about it. Some of the couples were childless, he found, because sexual intercourse was painful for them. He'd do simple things that would help them out, a hymenectomy, for example, or he'd take a tuck in the vaginal tissue so both husband and wife would obtain better sexual sensation. He just waded through endless numbers of little problems like that for people, straightening them out. Most general practitioners refused to pay any attention to such complaints, saying 'no thank you' to any suggestions that those were proper medical problems for doctors to have to deal with. Yet, those problems could be clear hell for the poor patients."

In the Rock household, familiarity with information about human sexuality was not equated with loose morals. Premarital sex was out of the question. "Why I . . . we [her sisters] would no more have gone to bed with somebody . . . it was absolutely out of the question," Rachel recalled. "Yet, if it did happen and I found myself pregnant out of wedlock, I knew that I could have told him and I would have been supported."

Although he once refused to prescribe the pill for an unmarried woman, Rock's private sexual views have modified considerably in recent years. During a visit with him he joked about the twin beds in the spare bedroom of his retirement home, a simple farmhouse in Temple, New Hampshire. "I let them [his grandchildren] do their own thing," he said with a shrug. "It no longer bothers me to think they might sleep with a friend. If they do happen to mate with the wrong partner, I just hope they don't hurry off and get married. Premarital sex doesn't hurt most level-headed young people if they act responsibly about it." By that, he meant, that they don't get pregnant when they are not ready to raise a child responsibly.

Neither Rock's extensive medical practice nor his research success ever brought him wealth, although many people thought that it had. After all, didn't the pill make millions for pharmaceutical companies? "They've got the wrong family," AJ once said. "That was simply not part of Daddy's ethic. I remember saying to him, 'For God's sake, Daddy, why don't you buy some stock?' Pincus is said to have made plenty, by buying stock in the company just before the break [FDA approval] was announced. We finally talked Daddy into buying one hundred shares of Searle stock. This was long after the pill was on the market. Then, he saw an article accusing him of exploiting women by 'experimenting' on them for financial gain. The stock was sold the next day."

Like him, his children follow the dictates of their conscience, an art in which they were well instructed. "Conscience is a very important thing, to all of us," Rachel says. "I grew up very aware of it, we all did. The daily conversation in our house was always full of little sayings, such as 'It doesn't matter whom you fool as long as you don't fool yourself.' "

Rock always thought through very carefully the philosophical implications of his work beforehand. He had a tremendous sense of curiosity and a passionate love for scientific discovery, his daughters say. "I think, in a very real sense, he felt that he had a contribution he could make to people . . . to humanity." Rachel said. "He doesn't think that the birth control pill was the most important thing he worked on. His work in reproductive physiology would be the most important, the largest contribution he made, when you think of how little people knew when he started and how much they know now. There is a time when you can rationalize that some area of research is right or wrong, but Daddy clearly went well beyond any fuzzy area in his thinking before he began. He's not stupid and he never undertook any research without considerable careful reasoning about its intent. We grew up as a Catholic family in a part of Boston that was largely Catholic. We were not very old when we knew that Daddy's relationship with the Church was strained at best because of the birth control issue," Rachel added. "I don't think that many of the local priests knew much about his research, however. By the late 1930s he already was attempting to get human eggs and sperm to unite *in vitro* . . . trying to achieve human conception in a glass dish. If they'd known about that, it really would have raised the hair on the back of their heads!"

3

PROBING HUMAN REPRODUCTION

THOSE who truly know the ins and outs of the story say that John Rock, and only John Rock, could have ushered the revolutionary birth control pill into the world on the scale and with the speed that it was done — virtually overnight on any historic timetable. Within a mere half-dozen years from the time the pill was first subjected to animal tests, it was being consumed daily by millions of women the world over. Never before in medical history had so monumental a discovery moved so rapidly and broadly into public use.

The fact that he was a deeply religious man, a superbly informed Catholic, with his own reasoned opinion of the pill's moral rightness, undoubtedly was a factor in its near universal acceptance by people of every faith the world over. That qualification, however, would not have sufficed had he not also been fully established as a medical specialist of great stature and as a research pioneer in the human reproductive process. In the mid to late 1950s when the pill was nearing its debut, Rock already was preeminent in his field. It was his name and his reputation that gave ultimate validity to the claims that the pill would protect women against unwanted pregnancy and do so to a remarkably reliable and safe degree.

By then, he'd spent three decades of his life trying to help women with the vexacious problems of not being able to have a baby or of having too many. His research reached into the very essence of the human life-begetting process. Original and ingeniously innovative, his work reflected a broad research interest that spanned the nature of the menstrual flow; the production, release, and character of the human fertile egg; the hormonal influences that hold sway over the female reproductive tract; and the still marvelously mysterious phenomenon of conception itself.

To appreciate the sweep of his thinking it is necessary to bear in mind how little was known about such matters when he began to explore them in 1925. Not until 1827 was the existence of the human female egg (ovum) discovered. Not until 1843 was it certain that the sperm actually enters the egg. Not until 1875 was it clearly demonstrated that human fertilization involves the *union* of the sperm nucleus with that of the ovum! The sex hormones that cycle a woman's fertility were not isolated until *after* Rock began his work; estrogen in 1929 and progesterone in 1934. Proof that all sex hormones, male and female, governing both sperm and egg development and timing their production, are themselves governed by still other hormones that come from the pituitary gland in the brain had come only in 1926. This revelation is still considered the most far-reaching discovery in reproductive biology, an electrifying breakthrough. The men who produced the first firm evidence of the pituitary gland's role as a remote control system in human reproduction, Selmar Aschheim and Bernard Zondek, later converted this knowledge into the first pregnancy test. Before that, there was none. In Rock's early research years, however, nothing was known about the first days and weeks of life for a human conceptus: the tiny packet of genetic material formed when human egg and sperm unite and from which every living person emerges.

Research tools were still primitive by today's standards. There were no electron microscopes, nor automated blood and chemistry tests, no antibiotics to combat contamination of specimens, and only poor sterilization equipment. Laboratories by and large were dingy, dreary, and dark. Rather than the steel and glass research palaces of today, Rock and his cohorts worked under conditions more similar to those depicted by Alec Guinness and *The Lavender Hill Mob.*

Yet Rock and many other scientific pioneers of the era more than made up in curiosity, ardor, and commitment what they lacked in equipment and funds. Despite the fact that research support seldom amounted to more than a few hundred to a few thousand dollars, opportunity for discovery was rife. Gynecology, as a medical specialty, was only fifty years old when Rock began his career, and had been limited largely to *treating* "diseases peculiar to women." The realm of human sexuality was very much still a "foreign" subject. In Europe, pioneers like Freud, Felix Adler, and Havelock Ellis were initiating explorations into the psychological and physical nature of human sexuality, but in the United States the subject was still anathema, a degrading and degenerate topic in most professional and social circles. Sexual intimacy did not frighten or disgust Rock. He later would say no one was a greater proponent of it than he. And he certainly was not dissuaded from studying and teaching human sexuality by the feigned virtue of others.

Rock had an invaluable advantage in the setting for his work, the Free Hospital for Women. Modeled after the New York Woman's Hospital, the first American institution of its kind, the Free was founded in 1875 and had as its first mission the curing of vesico-vaginal fistula, an abnormal opening between the bladder and vagina, a vicious and common complication of childbirth in that period. In 1925, when Rock's work was getting underway, the Free was ensconced on a four-acre lot, a beautiful riverside glen just upstream from Jamaica Pond in Brookline, a block away from Boston's city-line boundary. Constructed of yellow brick, the hospital was built in the style of a French estate house, gabled, turreted, dormered, and buttressed along the sides and rear with building-long pavillions in which patients could partake of fresh air and sunshine during long hospital stays. It had fifty beds, considered a lot for that era, along with modern X-ray equipment, and three operating rooms. Its founding fathers, early medical staff, and trustees were exceptionally dedicated, able, and foresighted. They assured the continued excellence of the hospital by forging an affiliation with Harvard Medical School; they devised the first recovery room for intensive postsurgical care of patients; they pioneered the medical application of Madame Curie's discovered radium for the treatment of cervical cancer; and they made provision for laboratories for research into the pathology of female disorders. Conceived as most of America's original hospitals were out of a noble mix of religious and medical philanthropy, the Free Hospital lived up to its name. Only poor women were entitled to its service and they could not be charged for hospital care, nor could the hospital's doctors charge a fee. Charitable contributions covered the patients' costs and doctors donated their time. Not until 1919 was the Parkway wing added to accommodate the growing number of well-to-do women who wanted access to the quality care that their poor sisters were receiving free.

The hospital attracted an elite coterie of gynecologists, among them many of Harvard's best qualified graduates. The staff was small but select. Most had trained at the Free and were imbued with its spirit of charitable care. An appointment to the staff at the hospital, however, virtually guaranteed a prized, monied private practice because the hospital's reputation was so superior. The Free also provided almost absolute research freedom, far less interference than at the larger, Harvard-affiliated hospitals in Boston proper. During Rock's scientifically bountiful years there, the Free became something of a private research preserve for its principal staffers, a cultured as well as competent clique of men also well versed in Harvard academic politics and content to remain aloof on their own protected turf. While medical insiders knew more or less what was going on in the research programs at the Free, the general public knew little of it.

During the first few years Rock established his basic practice as an obstetrician-gynecologist, practicing gynecology primarily at the Free, obstetrics at the Boston Lying-In Hospital; and both at the Mass. General Hospital. He also delivered babies at various other maternity hospitals and many at home, the most common setting for "confinement" until World War II. His initial appointment to the Harvard Medical School faculty was in 1922.

As the start of the 1930s, Rock was beginning what would be the most consuming interest of his research life: the tragic problem of infertility. He worked exclusively with human subjects, never animals, on both the clinical and research level simultaneously. If ways were to be found to help more childless couples to conceive, then clearly far more had to be known about exactly when conception took place and how pregnancy could be maintained.

He soon found that for a great many of the seemingly infertile couples who sought his help, the barrier was false modesty or the lack of even rudimentary information about sexual intercourse. He became marvelously adept at overcoming the reticence of sexually shy women and their needlessly embarrassed husbands. He first won their confidence with his genuine concern and friendliness. Then he conveyed the most explicit sex information, unabashedly. He managed it so well largely because of his utterly dignified manner, an ambassadorial sort of presence, that dispelled any suggestion of smuttiness or impropriety in the subject. At the patients' own level of understanding, he very plainly instructed them in robust, satisfying sex practices. His respectful courtesy was the key, and it carried over into his treatment of all women patients. Residents and interns learned from his example to remember that every woman was to be shown the respect and gentlemanly attendance due a lady. Rock personally called cabs for them, opened doors, offered them his arm. It restored their sense of dignity when they most needed it, after undergoing what they felt were humiliating gynecological examinations.

As with his infertile couples, Rock discovered that sexual ignorance also pervaded the medical profession. He soon expanded his individual counseling into full-scale lectures on sex relations which he gave to third- and fourth-year Harvard medical students. Any of them who came in snickering left the lecture hall chastened. The lectures were remarkable — direct, complete, specific, and remembered due to Rock's inimitable style of presenting the information, laced with a mischievous wit.

He customarily began with some pointed references to the "unbridled copulatory urge" of man's closest animal counterparts, monkeys and baboons. He then alluded to man's similar instincts that would be just as ruttily expressed, were it not for man's higher intellectual endowment and his capacity for love. While he preached loving monogamy and stressed the constant need for mutual respect and honor, he did not skirt the frank details. A young couple "in close proximal contact" he would begin, would find that the brain and conducting nerves "generate in the male an anxious but not unpleasant warmth, shall we say, in his penis, and in the female, an upsurge of affection. By both more intimate contact is sought, as sexual tension increases in the sex-pleasure cerebral centers and stirs a desirous sensitivity . . . that soon spreads to the female breasts while in the male, erection occurs, and with it an almost involuntary manual groping for responsive and further stimulating erogenous female zones. The girl's mounting emotion at last causes dilation of vessels in the vagina and clitoris, as tongue, lips and nipples are mutually stimulated, largely because of the male's penile-aggravated aggression." Spelling out in step-by-step terms the progression of the sex act, Rock would relate how finally, "the wet penis is slipped into the irresistible and non-resisting moistened vagina . . . in a final explosive coital release of aggrandized sex-togetherness-love tension!" He never neglected the prospect of pregnancy: "Now the two are parents — but can and will they supply their offspring with good parenthood? Otherwise, they have merely given their species a bit of raw material to float on the wings of chance." A complete run-down of known forms of contraception was presented with every lecture, though this violated Massachusetts' anti–birth control law, which prohibited even the dispensing of information.

Ironically, it was not the organized Catholic medical community that did anything to teach their women about "rhythm." Rock did. In the out-patient clinics at the Free Hospital for Women, he found so many poor Catholic women who were desperate to know about "rhythm," that he founded the first "rhythm" clinic in the United States and, perhaps, the world. Over the years from 1936 when it formally opened, thousands of women were personally instructed or discreetly mailed instruction in the method. Mrs. Elizabeth Snedeker, wife of Dr. Lendon Snedeker, the world-renowned physician-in-chief of Boston's Children's Hospital Medical Center, operated the Rhythm Clinic for Rock on an unpaid, volunteer basis for fourteen years.

The Rhythm Clinic was to pay unexpected dividends for the benefit of the infertile, though as a reliable method of contraception "rhythm" has dubious standing. Underlying the method was the independent discovery by Ogino and Knauss in the mid 1920s — that women are only fertile at midpoint in the menstrual cycle, when a woman's ovary expels an egg that is fertilizable if it encounters a male sperm. The hitch is that the specific day on which that event occurs is not certain but was generally estimated by Ogino and Knauss to occur between the twelfth and sixteenth day of the "average" twenty-eight-day menstrual cycle. Actually, the cycle later was shown to have a wide range, from twenty-two to thirty-two days, and in some cases even longer. The only overt clue to when ovulation is taking place is a slight drop in a woman's body temperature followed a day later by a sudden and sustained rise. To detect that subtle signal, a woman must keep a careful calendar check of her menstrual periods, take her temperature each morning before getting out of bed, and keep a record of both. After doing this for several months, a pattern of her fertile time of the month should emerge. If the couple refrains from sexual intercourse at that time, theoretically they are safe from pregnancy. The hazard is that many uncontrollable factors — illness, emotional upset, fatigue, and the like — can cause the timing of ovulation to vary. Women with a regular cycle might gamble on sex relations from day six to ten of the cycle, but to be absolutely safe, a couple would have to refrain from sexual intercourse until the temperature rise had occurred and stayed at that level for at least three days. For high-pregnancy-risk couples practicing rigorous rhythm, the time left for safe sexual relations could amount to little more than a week per month, at the end of the cycle. After years of collecting data on the cycles of women and tabulating the contraceptive effect of the rhythm method in women highly motivated to have it succeed, often because another pregnancy was life-threatening, Rock wrote it off in a classic report carried in the prestigious *New England Journal of Medicine.* If the stakes were high for the couple involved, "rhythm" was just too chancy to be recommended, he concluded. Besides, he did not feel that limited sex relations were enough to sustain the bond of marital love. He did not abandon the idea behind "rhythm," however, and pursued throughout his active research life ways to pinpoint ovulation. Neither he nor anyone else has yet fully succeeded. As some of his later research would show, the egg is only fertilizable for about twelve to twenty-four hours, the sperm potent for no more than forty-eight. If the day of ovulation could be accurately forecast, Rock believed many couples would choose to practice continence for the three days or so per month when conception *could* occur. It not only would be a natural, nonchemical, nonmechanical form of contraception attractive to many people, it also would be a method the Church could not oppose.

In Rock's hands, however, the data from the Rhythm Clinic was adroitly put to use to benefit infertile women. Applying the same information, turned inside out, he was able to guide marginally infertile women — or their husbands, when a low sperm count was the cause of the infertility — to concentrate their sex relations during the brief midcycle time when an egg was most likely to be ready and waiting. By so doing, hundreds of couples got the baby they so dearly desired with the help of a little "rhythm" practiced in reverse.

As early as 1930, Rock began to make his mark in the research world. Three reports that year under his sole authorship appeared in national medical and specialty journals.* He was already forty years old; a late-starter, but a man physically and psychologically geared for a long race. He paced himself like a long-distance runner. He was never hurried. His work style was characterized by unbounded energy but an energy expended at a studied and steady pace. He had a lightning mind, tempered by a passion for clarity and precision. He had a rare capacity for giving his full attention to the matter before him and then turning instantly to the next with the same concentration.

---

* They reflected his twin interest in obstetrics and infertility and were entitled "Progress in Obstetrics"; "Maternal Mortality: What Must Be Done About It"; and "Clinical Trials on the So-called Female Sex Hormones."

Colleagues observed that he behaved the same way when he relaxed, particularly at out-of-town meetings when he had no patients to worry about for a few days. On those occasions he often drank, danced, and cavorted socially well into the night. There is a legendary story of Rock at the elite Laurentian Hormone Conference of 1956 in Canada, treasured as a special memory by MGH gynecologist George S. Richardson. "Rock professed that he was bored with the whole idea of the regular banquet. This may have been a deliberate move on his part to escape from any discussion of oral contraceptives, but it was characteristic of Rock to seek and find what he called 'superior forms of entertainment.' Without much difficulty he persuaded a group of us to join him . . . and a rather retiring biochemist to drive us. At a neighboring establishment, we found just about the only other person in the dining room was a young man eating by himself. Rock proceeded to bear down on this young man in his usual manner — that of an actor trained in Shakespearean roles and drawing room comedies. Like everyone who has ever been confronted with this affable and yet grandiose presence, the young man was soon giving his personal psychological and sexual history. Before he knew it, Rock had persuaded him to join us and go on to another resort.

"At our next place there was not only a bar but also a capacious dance floor, which we all proceeded to enjoy under Rock's leadership. After cutting in on one couple, Rock came back with a detailed report of the sexual problems that these honeymooners were having and his recommendations, which were sure to 'clear the whole thing up.' His attempt to treat other honeymoon couples in similar fashion was soon modified by his discovery that many of the people were, as he put it, 'ladies and gentlemen of pleasure.' After all of us — and mostly Rock — enjoyed ourselves hugely, we returned again at breakneck speed to the Lodge. Those who were still talking science on the lawn under the stars were regaled by our evening's finale — the sight of our party plunging nude into the swimming pool." Even more amazing was Rock's appearance bright-eyed and ready to go again at seven the next morning, when the scientific sessions opened at breakfast.

There is a terrible rivalry in science as in other academic fields. The sniping goes on covertly and under the guise of an interest solely in the purity of the work. Money, though important, is not the main motive. It is the demon Fame that occasionally reduces even the most eminent scientists to petty backbiting and spiteful little slanders. At

Harvard the method, carried out with great finesse, was to damn with faint praise. Not even best friends rise above it. In that competitive milieu, Rock had surprisingly few detractors. Yet, it is interesting that in thirty-five years of annual reports of the operations of the Free Hospital for Women not once is Rock's work paid a compliment, not even when he and his colleagues made spectacular discoveries. When the pill was approved and Rock exalted by the news media, no notice is given except one comment that the work of others was not of the sort that attracted "publicity." Everybody in the Harvard inner circle got the point.

It is true that a great deal of Rock's research work was carried out with others, but his research partners credit him with conceiving nearly all the projects and for handling critical aspects of the studies. Along with a handful of collaborators from the senior staff of the Free Hospital, Rock attracted a flock of young research fellows, some two hundred of them over the years. All were anxious to work for a pittance just to be permitted to work at his side. He always prominently credited them on research papers, knowing the importance of getting their names established early. They came from around the globe to his laboratory, from Greece, Turkey, Japan, India, Sweden, Italy, France, Germany, Great Britain, and a number from Central and South America. In time Rock's fellows became outposts of his philosophy, promoting birth control programs in their native countries.

He often brought them along with him to scientific meetings to introduce them to the leading figures in obstetrics and gynecology and in government funding centers who might advance their budding careers. To mask his generosity, Rock would justify their accompanying him on such jaunts by contending they were needed in case he took ill while traveling. He also did what he could to pad out their pay on the pretext they were teaching him a foreign language or some similar ruse. He was very fond and very fatherly toward the young men who came to his laboratory, mindful of his own financial hardships as a young resident. He would have them to dinner at his home and serve them some good roast beef and Yorkshire pudding to boost their spirits. There, they would talk long into the night, debating fine points of ethics and philosophy, as well as science. Many of them became his surrogate sons, especially Dr. Celso-Ramon Garcia and Luigi Mastroianni. (Mastroianni now is the William Goodell Professor and Chairman of the Department of Obstetrics and Gynecology and Garcia is the William Shippen, Jr. Professor and Director of the Division of Human Reproduction at the University of Pennsylvania School of Medicine.) Both worked with Rock at the make-or-break time when the pill was being tested. Garcia eventually played a role nearly as large as that of Rock and Pincus.

Those outside the inner research circle of the Free Hospital provide another measure of Rock's work. One of the country's most distinguished gynecologic endocrinologists, Dr. Janet McArthur, a member of the Harvard Medical School faculty and co-director of the Vincent Memorial Laboratory at MGH, has more reason than most to be discriminating in her view, for she nearly succeeded him as director of his final bastion, the famed, independent Rock Reproductive Research Center. McArthur, a splendid researcher in her own right and a conservative woman not given to overstatement, says unequivocally, "He was way ahead of his time. His research crackled with originality. You would constantly marvel at the fertility of his mind and the breadth of his thinking. He could see the potential pertinence in the most remote information. He had great daring and courage and was an altogether brave man."

Rock's laboratory genius was in taking what was known, plus what was available, and then by asking different questions of the material, to discover new answers. One of his early feats was to date the characteristics of the endometrium, the lining of the womb, that changed in accordance with the days of a woman's menstrual cycle. Until then, each time a specimen of the tissue lining of the womb was obtained for examination, a measure of how normal (or abnormal) its appearance was could only be roughly gauged according to the status of many components of the tissue or the glands and blood vessels in it. The process was very cumbersome and nonspecific. Yet the exact time in the cycle that the endometrial tissue looked one way or another could reveal whether a woman could and did ovulate — or not. The appearance of the tissue also told whether the hormone governance of the cycle progressed on schedule, or whether the tissue was right for one phase of her cycle, but very wrong for another. Late in the 1930s, Dr. George Smith called Rock's attention to a curetting (a sample of tissue scraped from the lining of the womb with an instrument called a curette). Smith estimated it was a specimen of about the twenty-first day of the cycle. The question arose in Rock's mind: could all curettings be *described* by dates?

Rock already had devised a far less painful way to obtain curettings. Instead of drawing segments of tissue from the womb back through the neck of the womb, with a cutting and pinching device, Rock used a twin-tubed instrument, fitted with a curbed and hooded blade at the end of one canal, and the other an open tube. This way he could obtain sizable slices of the tissue and aspirate (use suction) them back "without appreciable bleeding or pain" to the patient. His aspiration technique became the accepted method of choice. Using it, he and Dr. Marshall K. Bartlett, a resident intern at the Free Hospital under Rock's tutelage in 1938 (and later a distinguished surgeon at MGH) collected hundreds of samples of endometrial tissue, taken for biopsy study. They got others from staff surgeons. By noting ten or so qualities of the tissue, they gradually found they could correlate the tissue appearance to the day in the menstrual cycle. From then on, doctors could discuss the condition and sequences of womb tissue by date alone. "Elaborate descriptions were no longer needed," Rock pointed out; "a simple day numeral gave the whole picture."

Rock overlooked nothing in his search to pin down the time of ovulation. In the late 1930s, he was the first in the country to look into changes in the electrical potential of the female vagina as an indicator that a woman was ovulating. Two basic scientists at Yale had first discerned such electric potential change., — from negative to positive and back again — in vaginal tissue in rabbits. In some quarters, the swings in the electric potentials were being interpreted as signifying that a woman ovulated more than once a cycle. With the help of an electro-physiologist, James M. Snodgrass, Rock spent three years trying to find out whether the shift signified ovulation at all in women, his primary concern.

To prove — or disprove, as it turned out — the significance of the electrical potential, Rock wired up willing patients at the most propitious time of their monthly cycle. The subjects were women awaiting surgery at the Free. Whatever the hour of day or night that their electric potential changed, he would operate immediately. It drove the nurses crazy being called out of bed to prep the patients and assist in the operating room at three o'clock in the morning, if that was when the electric potential looked prime. But they adored Rock, so they went along with it. The tests were disappointing for Rock's purposes. They proved only that the electrical difference recorded in the tissue surfaces were just that — surface differences — not ovulation. His suspicion that the electrical changes reflected hormone changes, however, was confirmed years later by others with far more sophisticated equipment. So far as Rock was concerned, the 1939 final results were important, because they at least "stopped a pernicious heresy concerning ovulation time."

The notion became popular in the 1940s, that adopting a baby seemed to "cure" some cases of infertility. Often, or so it appeared, as soon as the barren couple took home an adopted baby, the wife became pregnant. It was theorized that having a baby in their care somehow overcame the adoptive parents' nervousness about producing one on their own. They became more "relaxed" and the next thing they knew, they found they weren't sterile after all. From Rock's understanding of the intricacies of infertility, he doubted the "adoption syndrome" was true. So during the late 1940s he and one of his research fellows, Dr. Fred Hanson undertook a study of the effect of adoption on subsequent fertility. From several adoption agencies, they obtained the names of two hundred adopting parents and as much of the marital background and physical findings as they could. They contacted the parents by questionnaire, dropping from the group those in whom the husband or wife were anatomically provably sterile. "So we ended up with seventy couples in whom stress could be a factor," Rock explained. "However, in only 6 percent of these cases was there an indication that improvement of emotional tone in the wife following adoption might have been a factor in the pregnancies which followed. We were unable to demonstrate that adoption had any therapeutic effect on infertility." Nonetheless, the myth persisted. In the mid-1960s, the National Institute of Health funded a much larger study, undertaken by Rock with Dr. Christopher Tietze, then of the National Committee on Maternal Health, New York, and Helen McLaughlin of the Boston Children's Service Association. This time 249 inexplicably barren adopting parents were compared with 113 similarly infertile nonadopting couples. At the time it was generally assumed that there was a spontaneous cure rate of 6 to 8 percent in adopting couples and 10 percent in nonadopting couples. This study, however, disclosed a 35 percent cure rate in the nonadopting and 26 percent of the adopters. Again, adoption had not improved the likelihood of spontaneous pregnancy.

The far higher incidence of pregnancies in the second study was attributed to the long-term payoff in medical and counseling that couples in both groups had received two years prior to the study. Once again Rock had cleared the air and put to rest what he called "the widespread idea that mental tension interferes with fertility, *in spite of regular ovulation, adequate coitus and good insemination*." The studies were very "ticklish" propositions, however, because adoption is supposed to be a secret affair. Indeed when they started (in 1940) one of the agencies promptly withdrew its cooperation. They had received a letter from one of the adoptive parents threatening to sue them for invasion of privacy. As always, Rock made use of information gained from the study for purposes beyond what was originally intended: by becoming acquainted with adoption agencies all over the world, he became able to refer hopelessly sterile couples to those agencies where he had personal contacts.

In recognition of his extensive clinical and research work in the field of human ovulation, Rock was chosen by the *New England Journal of Medicine,* the foremost medical journal in the world, to write the definitive article on ovulation in 1941. It was carried in the magazine's Medical Progress Section. Rock was asked to repeat that virtuoso performance for the same publication in 1949, this time updating what was currently known about the "Physiology of Human Conception." In that presentation, he begins in his literate style with the observation: "Although simple parthenogenesis [self-fertilization] is not at all uncommon in invertebrates — for instance in ants and bees — it does not, as far as is known, occur in human beings, who must produce eggs and sperm and then effect their conjugation." In the report, Rock elected to deal strictly with the physical "aspects of this complicated process since the beguiling psychologic motivation and mechanisms lie in a mixture of too much fancy with too little fact." Ten years later, he, along with Celso-Ramon Garcia, who worked cheek-by-jowl with Rock and Pincus on the pill, would co-author with Rock's assistant Miriam Menkin, for presentation in the annals of the prestigious New York Academy of Sciences, "A Theory of Menstruation," a subject given little serious scientific attention by a male-dominated medical world. In elegant language all too rare in science articles, he elucidated the wondrous, cyclic life-and-death of the lining of the female womb; its preparation to receive and nurture new life if it is conceived; the manner in which all the life-supporting systems are marshaled "for timely service to aspiring spermatazoa but surely in dutiful expectation of the kingly (or queenly) morula [the fertilized egg] should it arrive." If that does not happen, he wrote with a tinge of sadness of the subsequent retrenchment, there occurs the thinning and buckling of the glands and lining of the womb, the squeezing down and narrowing of tiny blood vessels, and the final death and disruption of the intended womb. The inevitable bleeding begins, "menstruation has occurred," he notes, "and will soon be evident to disturb the woman (or comfort her, as the case may be)." In other reports on menstruation he clarified the use of hormones to relieve premenstrual tension and pain, which he never dismissed as emotional or self-indulgent female complaints as did many gynecologists.

He even came to the rescue of women who were accused of using tampons for masturbatory or other sexual diversions. In a 1965 study, he dealt directly with the misbegotten issue, pulling no punches: "The allegation that morality may be affected by tampons seems unwarranted because [there are no] nerve endings in the deep vaginal mucosa [lining.] A soft cotton tampon has no properties which would make it suitable as a dildo. The English female physician P. H. Gosling has commented that only those curiously ignorant of female physiology would regard the tampon as a contrivance for sexual pleasure. The vagina in fact is part of the region which [Dr. J. R.] Goodall [of Montreal] has so aptly described as 'the great silent area of the pelvis.' " Rock wrote, the tampon was "being implicated in defloration and masturbation," thus confronting some ecclesiastics and sexually pristine physicians at the time who were preoccupied with the possibility that tampons were affording women some secret, naughty pleasures (and suspecting the same of jockey shorts in men). All in all, he reassured the worriers that tampons "have no deleterious effects,* physiologically, clinically, or *morally*."

Even though he was achieving spectacular success with infertile patients by 1956 — achieving an astonishing cure rate of 30 percent — he was not satisfied. "One takes satisfaction in knowing people, overfertile people, whom you've spared another child," he said in 1980, "but I think about . . . I dwell more, even now [at age 90] on the failures. It's gratifying to be mindful of the number of infertile women you helped have a child, but they're not the ones I remember. No . . . I remember those I failed."

If they were to be helped three obstacles had to be overcome. One was "obstruction in the oviducts" (the Fallopian tubes that connect the egg-bearing ovaries to the nest of the womb), "a common complete, and hitherto discouraging cause of sterility," Rock wrote in 1951. The

---

* Rock's report responded primarily to moralistic objections to tampon use. Safety was a secondary consideration. Further, tampons of 1965 were less absorbent, and not anatomically shaped to create the kind of reservoir now suggested to be associated with toxic shock syndrome.

second was insufficient number of good sperm in a particular mating, and the third major barrier to pregnancy was an under- or nonfunctioning ovary. Rock made major research contributions to all three problems.

With the late Dr. William Mulligan, an esteemed Free Hospital gynecological surgeon, Rock developed a succession of surgical maneuvers to try to open, clear, or reconstruct the oviducts, the passageway from ovary to womb. With Charles Easterday, a young surgical resident, they introduced new synthetic materials, polyethylenes that were firm, nonadhesive, and permitted blood vessel growth, as replacements for the damaged tubes. The synthetic also was used as a tunnel to hold the tubes open while healing. Earlier, inert metals, such as silver, were temporarily inserted to serve as wedges to keep the tubes open with little success.

The Fallopian tubes, twin, flexible, trumpet-shaped tubes, are a mere four and a half inches long, with an inner passageway only a fraction of an inch in diameter. The wedges and polyethylene implants (first tried in 1947) had to be comparably tiny in size. To avoid undue injury to the delicate tube, Rock and Mulligan "gradually included in our operating kit, instruments commonly used by neurosurgeons and vascular surgeons" — a very early move toward microsurgery.

Rock tried tuboplasty (as it is technically called) on hundreds of desperate patients, among them the obscure and the famous. One was Merle Oberon, the leading English actress of the day. When Merle was sixteen or seventeen years old her mother had had both of Merle's tubes severed and a portion of them removed. She was a young star, an ingenue, and her mother didn't want her career interfered with by an inadvertent pregnancy. Years later when she was desperate to have a child, Merle went first to a gynecologist in New York, who transplanted one ovary directly into the uterus. That couldn't work at all, of course, since the fertilized egg must spend four days traversing the tube. If the timing is even one day off, too slow or too fast, the conception is lost, and for a conception to succeed, fertilization must take place in the tube to begin with. "The New York doctor's efforts only made conditions worse," Rock vividly recalled, "leaving scar tissue all over the place, which we took out. She was the first one I used silver probes on to try to keep the reconstructed canals open. But it couldn't work. The other doctor hadn't left anything to work with, the tubal tissue was nearly absent. She would have been the happiest girl in the world if she could have become pregnant, but there was absolutely nothing that could be done."

In the arena of artificial insemination, Rock was among the earliest pioneers. He became expert in the parameters of adequate and inadequate sperm count; sperm physiology and behavior; the biochemical climate in the female that enhanced sperm potency; and finally, the techniques for freezing and storing sperm. Again, with Garcia (and the editorial aid of Miriam Menkin) Rock produced a landmark two-article series for the specialty journal *Fertility and Sterility* in 1946 on "Refrigerant Preservation of Human Spermatazoa." The work, begun six years earlier, revealed that the speed with which sperm are frozen or thawed is less important in their recovery and viability than is the freshness of the sperm at the outset. Sperm frozen for six months, they also found, survived just as well as those frozen only a month. The advantage to the infertile is that men with low sperm counts can have their sperm frozen and banked so that a more potent concentration can be pooled with which to impregnate their wives.

In the mid 1960s, when he was approaching seventy-five, Rock was still chipping away at the final obstacle for the woman whose sterility was due to her ovulating irregularly or not at all for no known reason. Others had begun testing new compounds aimed at prodding the pituitary gland in the brain to turn on and up the production of estrogen to nudge the ovary into ripening an egg. With Dr. Robert Kistner of the Boston Hospital for Women and two research fellows, Rock was among the first to apply the new fertility drugs, experimentally. Rock's long experience with the fundamentals of ovulation and its vagaries were key to the 1964 study. Using a new compound, clomiphene citrate, they tried various doses and various lengths of treatment. Rock relied on an updated version of a "rhythm" chart with its telltale temperature shift to detect whether ovulation occurred. Eight of the thirty-six volunteer patients became pregnant and in twenty-one more there was proof they had, indeed, finally ovulated. More than that, the study refined the use of clomiphene, indicating that it was most effective when given in moderately high doses and selectively on the eighth to eleventh day of the menstrual cycle. "Clomiphene," their report concluded, "offers *exceptional* promise as a . . . preparation which appears to induce ovulation in selected cases of ovulatory failure." A new era in the treatment of infertility was established.

Kistner, who had been another of Rock's research fellows, still remembers the first time he saw Rock, when Rock was addressing the American Gynecological Society. "He was such a stately, handsome man, impeccably dressed in a gray suit, dark tie and with that magnificent white hair. He looked like God himself standing there. No matter what he said, you'd believe it, but it was all true. He did far more to move gynecology ahead than any other single figure in the field. He was the most essentially kind man I've ever known, yet exhilarating and stimulating. Did I like him? I loved him!"

One of Rock's pet contentions was that nature somehow arranged, as a species survival mechanism, for men and women to be most sexually attracted to one another at the time of greatest fertility. Only something like that, he felt, could explain the frequency of conception against overwhelming odds. By 1959, entomologists had shown that substances called pheromones exist in insects and give off a sexually alluring smell. Rock wondered if such pheromones were also present in humans. His interest was further piqued by the postulations of psychiatrists that such smells played a role in the sexual development of children. During the Oedipal period, the psychiatric hunch held, the child might be attracted by the odor of the parent of the opposite sex and repulsed by the odor of the ipsisexual (same sex) parent. With his research fellow Jacqueline Scoal Vierling, Rock set out to test the idea of odor as a sexual attractant and whether it was strongest when a woman is most fertile.

Using Exaltolide, a musky, he-man odorant used as a base in perfume, Rock and Vierling tested seventy-three female student nurses to see if they were more sensitive to the smell when they were ovulating and therefore most receptive to pregnancy. The nurses not only were supersensitive to the Exaltolide odor precisely at the time ovulation was due, they again were similarly sensitive on precisely the eighth day before the onset of menstruation. Nothing — not smoking, medications, respiratory infections, or room temperature — dampened the keenness of their awareness of the musky smell at those two times in the monthly cycle. Those are the two days of peak levels of estrogen in the cycle.

Because nasal tissue in women is a secondary target for the female hormone estrogen, it would be present to a high degree in the lining of the nose whenever it is high in their sex organs. Theoretically, that could explain the dramatic twice-monthly smell sensitivity of the nurses — and probably all women — to the manly odor of musk. While Rock's study only scratched the surface of the possibility of human pheromones, it nonetheless showed that many subtle sex attractants probably exist about which next to nothing is known. Undoubtedly, they are at play in human sex relations, as Rock had surmised.

Even after the pill was born, Rock continued to hunt for other, simple contraceptives. Knowing as he did the intricate conditions that must prevail for egg and sperm to form, reach one another and unite with exquisite timing, he looked for a way to throw just one factor off course. As a potential male contraceptive, he thought heat might do it. It has long been known that in men, as in most animals, sperm production is highly sensitive to temperature changes. The minuscule, tadpole-shaped male spermatazoon is many times smaller than the female egg. In fact, a sperm is the smallest of all human cells and the egg, the largest. Sperm form and mature in twin glands, the testes, that lie within the pouched testicles of the scrotum. Normally, a healthy young man emits 200 million to 300 million sperm with each ejaculate at sexual climax. Below 60 million, a man is considered functionally sterile. The scrotum normally is a trifle cooler than the body because sperm production is more efficient at a marginally lower temperature. If the scrotum is chilled — or heated — beyond its optimum temperature, sperm production drops quickly and markedly. The man with a marginally low sperm count, who take a long, hot tub before retiring, unwittingly may sterilize himself, temporarily. If that is his daily routine, he will prolong the sterilizing effect.

For a number of years, Rock tried to find a practical way to cool or warm the scrotum just beyond the normal temperature range, with two purposes in mind. First, he hoped that by resting the sperm-production of the testes he might get a rebound effect that would step up sperm production when the temperature again was normalized. That way he hoped to boost the sperm count in men with borderline infertility. As always, however, he also saw the potential for contraception in the same maneuver — used in reverse. In a series of studies with Garcia and research fellows Eliot Rivo and Derek Robinson, Rock's hunch again proved to be on target. Sperm production was lowered to 10 percent of normal — well below the sterile mark — by warming the scrotum. And, as he predicted, the sperm count skyrocketed when normal temperatures were restored.

It was relatively easy to produce the sterilizing-fertilizing effect in the laboratory merely by exposing the scrotums of male volunteers to a heat-emitting light bulb. But it was a tricky business trying to find a way to do it in an aesthetically acceptable way for men going about the course of their daily lives. Rock came up with an oilcloth liner, backed by Kleenex to prevent chafing, that was worn inside ordinary jockey shorts or an athletic supporter. The gear was soon dubbed a scrotal muff, or the Rock-strap. "A simple modification in modern clothing may provide a burgeoning population with an easy method of fertility control," Rock said, "and the importance of such . . . is not be gainsaid." A continually hot scrotum, however, hasn't much appeal, it seems, for the masses.

Light, Rock thought, held similar universal potential as a contraceptive for women. It was an elusive concept, but it had a kernel of insight. Studies by Richard Wurtman at Massachusetts Institute of Technology have shown that light is centrally involved in human circadian rhythms, the biological clocks that time the ebb and flow of hormones and cycle body chemistry. Light also is well known to influence reproduction in animals. Phenemonally, it is the increased amount of daylight in springtime that triggers ovulation in sheep and other farm animals, as well as birds. In humans, the first clue to the reproductive role of light was discovered thirty years ago by Elizabeth Zacharias, also of MIT. Paradoxically, she showed that blind girls begin to menstruate at an earlier age than the sighted, due to deprivation of light signals to the brain. The earlier menarche stems from the fact that other mechanisms switch on earlier in these girls because they escape the restraint of and supersede light-sensitive factors. In rats, because they are nocturnal animals, the reverse is true: constant exposure to light stops ovulation completely.

In 1967, with the help of a theoretical physicist, Edmond Dewan, Rock studied fourteen women who agreed to sleep for four nights at midcycle with a 100-watt light bulb burning near their beds. While the results are totally inconclusive, they are marginally suggestive that the women's menstrual patterns became more uniform and regular. That effect, however, could easily be due to other psychological factors. Yet the influence of light in human reproduction still cannot be easily dismissed. Newer studies by Wurtman at MIT in 1975 found that there is a daily rhythm to the rate at which humans excrete a hormone, melatonin, produced in the pineal, the master-gland in the brain. Melatonin's production is directly influenced by alterations in light exposure. In all animals and birds, melatonin induces sleep, *inhibits ovulation*, and hastens sexual maturation. It would be remarkable if humans were not somehow affected, though more subtly. Rock's idea may yet be redeemed.

Throughout all of Rock's research, the single, most compelling need was to find a way to predict a day or two in advance exactly when ovulation would occur. Not only would it have solved the greatest obstacle to contraception, it became of vital importance to his attempts to fertilize a human egg in the laboratory and to the collecting of early-stage embryos. Before Rock and his two associates did the work, no one had ever seen the beginnings of human life, not to mention created it.

4

THE HUMAN EGG HUNT

THE most wondrous of all phenomena, the transmission of life itself, does not begin with the birth of a newborn baby. It starts a generation earlier when the parents are born and culminates with spectacular drama when conception occurs as it does, within a warm, moist translucent, shell-pink tube, undulating to and fro all the while. The odds by which one egg out of a potential half-million is fertilized by one sperm out of potential billions, on a timetable highly subject to chance, are totally incalculable. Each union is a biological miracle. It was in that virtually unexplored arena that Rock elected to probe for new insight into the origin of human life.

At the moment of birth each tiny female infant already carries within her the germ cells of her children to be. In twin, almond-shaped ovaries lie the seeds, so to speak, of a half-million reproductive eggs, called oocytes. They remain dormant until puberty. Even then, over the thirty-five-year span of her fertility from menarche to menopause, only about five hundred of the half-million will be called forth. Each month, a handful will be brought to the brink of ripening, but only one will burst free of its fluid-filled bed and begin the immense journey toward a possible encounter with a sperm and potential new life. The egg will be receptive to mating for only twelve hours. Cumbersome in size in contrast to submicroscopic sperm, the free egg is picked up by the fringe-like extensions of the entryway to the Fallopian tube and moved inside (about an inch) by tidelike motions of the tube. There, the egg's destiny is decided. It will be impregnated by a sperm, or not.

The male infant is born with its potential for parenthood already present, too. Within the twin testes lie glands, lined with stem cells, from which fertilizing sperm will arise following puberty. Thereafter, by the billion, male sperm is generated on a sixty-four-day cycle. The constant renewal of the supply must be relieved every few days by bursts, ejaculations, of 300-or-more million sperm at a time. The tad-pole-shaped sperm have to win out over enormous adversities if one is to reach and rendezvous with a female egg. In the female reproduc-tive tract, the chemical climate is favorable only at midcycle. There, the final step in sperm maturation takes place if conditions are right. Fe-male secretions trigger chemical chain reactions that cause sperm to shed a protective hood, baring a sheath that will imbed instantly upon contact with an egg's surface. Once past that preparatory step, ana-tomical barriers must be overcome. The sperm must propel itself through the entrance to the cervix into and across the pear-shaped womb, past the gateway into the Fallopian tubes, and along two-thirds of its length. It is the longest and most arduous journey of life. Sperm have but a forty-eight-hour life in which to run this obstacle course. If an egg is waiting, only one sperm will succeed.* Within a split second, the egg cell will become impregnable to all others.

In 1938 Rock embarked on two intertwined lines of research into the phenomenon of conception; research that stands among the great landmarks in medical science. One was conception of human life in a test tube. The other, the retrieval of the earliest specimens of human life ever seen. The "egg hunt" as the work was dubbed, went on for fifteen years. Over the course of the project, some thousand eggs were garnered from women surgical patients who were undergoing hysterec-tomies, having their womb, Fallopian tubes, and ovaries removed. As scientific feats, the two lines of research remain all the more remark-able for the old-fashioned conditions under which they were achieved. It is doubly ironic that advances in early detection of pregnancy rule out any prospect that the work will ever be repeated.

There was nothing fancy about the equipment or the laboratories where Rock and his colleague, pathologist Arthur Tremain Hertig,

---

* Rare exceptions occur, of course, accounting for multiple births, when more than one egg ripens simultaneously, or more than one sperm penetrates at exactly the same instant.

were to search for already fertilized human eggs: Hertig's on the ground floor of the Parkway wing of the Free Hospital for Women and Rock's on the third. But the procedures they set up for obtaining the eggs were ingenious, and Rock and Hertig, along with Rock's indefatigable assistant Miriam Menkin, were singularly resourceful.

By happenstance, all three were moving into the Harvard orbit during the mid-1930s and had been peripherally involved in human egg work — along with Gregory Pincus whose work would lead to the development of "the pill." Back then, Pincus had started looking for human eggs, as a sideline to other research he had under way while studying for his doctorate in science at Harvard University and later as a junior member of the biology faculty. Miriam Menkin had worked for a bit as one of Pincus's assistants. Hertig was completing his residency training in pathology at the (then) Boston Lying-In Hospital, Harvard's principal maternity center.

Rock and others from the Free Hospital occasionally sent ovarian tissue over to Pincus on the Cambridge campus, to see if he could locate any burgeoning eggs in it. Rock and Pincus experimented with various techniques to see if the elusive human eggs could be winnowed from the tissue, but none succeeded. Hertig was doing the same thing at the Lying-In. At that stage, however, all their efforts were only desultory and the probing was further hampered by the lack of any timing in regard to the ovulatory phase of the ovarian segments: if an egg were ripening, it was wholly by chance. Had any been found, Pincus was not in a position to attempt test-tube fertilization. He had no access to fresh sperm, and besides, his laboratory was geared to basic animal research. He did the groundwork, however, and in time succeeded outstandingly by fertilizing rabbit eggs in a test tube and in implanting them in pre-primed female rabbits. Pincus learned that nearly ripe rabbit eggs could be "matured" by incubating them overnight in rabbit blood. Later, Rock and Miriam Menkin would capitalize on that discovery.

When the "egg hunt" began in 1938, Arthur Hertig, who later became an eminent scientist in his own right, was only a young man. He had come to the Free Hospital by a somewhat circuitous route, but one that would pay big dividends in harvesting human eggs. Born in Minnesota in 1904, he had started out to be an entomologist, a researcher in the field of insect studies that relate to human diseases, as was his older brother, Marshall. While working on a summer research project in China with Marshall in 1926, Hertig met Dr. David Edsall, then dean of Harvard Medical School. As a result, Hertig transferred from the University of Minnesota, where he was a second-year medical student, to Harvard. The next break came, as Hertig sees it, when he met Dr. S. Burt Wolbach, chairman of pathology at HMS, and already famous for his work on the rickettsiae organisms in typhus fever.* Wolbach swerved Hertig's medical interest to pathology. Just as Hertig was completing his residency training in pathology, the Lying-In Hospital decided to start a formal pathology lab. Hertig got the job of resident pathologist there in 1931. He had no particular interest at that time in obstetric pathology, but a paying position in the Depression year of 1931 was not to be passed up. Although colleagues warned him there was no future in obstetrical pathology because childbirth was a "normal phenomenon," he soon came to appreciate the many dire pathological problems of pregnancy. With the discovery of antibiotics still many years in the future, childbed fever (puerperal sepsis) was still a frequent killer, as was toxemia, the dangerous late-in-pregnancy complication marked by high blood pressure, excessive weight gain, and fluid retention, often a prelude to deadly convulsions and coma (eclampsia). These became special research interests of Hertig's, as did infant mortality and spontaneous abortion. To master the field fully, he became board certified in obstetrics and gynecology, a highly unusual step. In the course of his research career, he did much of the classic work on the hydatidiform mole, a most peculiar, sometimes deadly, pre-cancerous cluster of cysts that may form from residual placental tissue in the womb; and on carcinoma-in-situ of the cervix, pre-cancerous changes of tissue in the neck of the womb. Such changes didn't exist for the pathologist prior to 1939 and Hertig's studies.

His unique preparation for the egg hunt, however, grew out of special research he undertook in 1933. He won a National Research Fellowship with the great human embryologist, Dr. George L. Streeter, at the Carnegie Institution of Washington in Baltimore, Maryland. While, there, Hertig worked out the details of how the monkey — and the human — placenta forms its own blood supply. Flaws in that process, he found, were a major underlying factor in spontaneous abortion. Hertig also learned from some of the institution's leading scientists the techniques they were developing for finding fertilized eggs in primates

---

* Rickettsiae are infectious agents which are intermediate between viruses and bacteria and which are passed to humans by ticks, fleas, lice, and mites. Rickettsiae are familiar to most people as the cause of Rocky Mountain spotted fever.

(rhesus monkeys) very similar to man. One of the advantages with primates was that the hunt for the fertilized eggs could be timed to coincide with the time they mated.

Fortuitously, Hertig was appointed pathologist at the Free in 1938, in tandem with his appointment at the Boston Lying-In. Rock was the only other person to also hold such joint appointments at both those hospitals. Hertig and Rock, thus, were cast together in an ideal position to take up the egg hunt in earnest. Both were, as Pincus had been, at least in part inspired by Aldous Huxley's futuristic shocker, *Brave New World*. In that 1932 novel, human eggs were fertilized, grown, and hatched in a laboratory and pre-selected to develop as workers and masters. "We'd all started it, ineffectually," Hertig remembered. "Pincus was primarily interested as a fundamental biologist. Rock's interest was the fertility aspect and the fundamental physiology, as was mine. No one knew what a human embryo looked like during the first two weeks of life, nor exactly when conception took place, or where, and nothing was known about when or how the young conceptus implanted in the lining of the womb." Hertig is not certain whose idea the egg hunt was. "Brain children are a lot like regular children. Sometimes it's hard to determine legitimacy. But it was John [Rock] who was the motivating spirit as far as using clinical material [patients] was concerned. In our original hit-or-miss efforts [with Pincus] we looked at an enormous amount of eggs that weren't eggs, just cellular debris, because none of us had seen an early fertilized human egg. The heartaches and the pitfalls were very real because the art of actually recognizing a human egg hadn't been mastered. We'd washed out lots of oviducts [Fallopian tubes] and found a lot of stuff that we realized later on were not eggs but little bits of the lining of the tubes. These were artifacts in the sense that they were rolled up little balls of tissue that looked like early fertilized eggs. When we finally did find a specimen that really was an embryo, we immediately knew it was the real thing. It's like anything else that's genuine. Once you see it, there's not very much doubt."

Timing was the keystone to success; the single most critical element. Groping for eggs in any old specimens of ovarian or tubal tissue on a hit-or-miss basis was too blind an approach. It was too wasteful to spend time looking for something that probably wasn't there to begin with. But by 1938 Rock had a few years experience with his rhythm clinic patients and had established a beachhead of knowledge about women's ovulatory time. Hertig was well aware from his Carnegie Institution studies that the secret to finding fertilized monkey eggs was to correlate the search with copulation at the most opportune ovulation time. But how could this be done with people? Women could hardly be set to copulating on schedule and then subjected to sterilizing surgery merely to assure Hertig and Rock more promising tissue samples in which they would have a better chance of finding a human conceptus.

Rock conceived of a way to go about it, however. He started at the opposite end of the puzzle, with women who needed hysterectomies for valid medical reasons. They were going to lose their wombs anyway. The strategem he envisioned was to time their surgery so that it coincided with ovulation, or shortly thereafter. Possibly, just possibly, they might also be in a very early, indeterminable stage of early pregnancy.

Even as Rock had begun to use the rhythm method in reverse to aid fertility, he saw a way to also put it to use for the egg hunt. It was very "iffy," but it just might work. If women awaiting hysterectomies kept rhythm charts to gauge when they were most likely to ovulate . . . and if they kept track during the month before surgery of when and if they had sexual intercourse with their husbands . . . and if that intercourse coincided with ovulation . . . Then, if surgery were performed shortly thereafter, the odds on finding a fertilized egg would be markedly better.

It unquestionably was a delicate ethical maneuver. Both Rock and Hertig thought about the ethical implications long and hard. Eventually, for both, it came down to "a necessary scientific endeavor using material that would have gone to waste but would not have been put to the use for which the Lord intended it." Neither Rock nor Hertig considered the conceptuses they hoped to find to be abortuses. At the few days to two or so weeks of development of the fertilized eggs, Hertig and Rock considered them undifferentiated bits of protoplasm, tiny gelatinous packets of human protein, destined to end up, undetected, in a surgical waste bin.

Admittedly, most of the volunteer patients were Catholics. They were all "free" patients receiving treatment at the Free Hospital's gynecology clinic. "I can tell you that they were hand picked and they were treated with tender loving care. They regarded themselves, once they were in the study, as very special, private patients. They were operated on by Dr. Rock himself. I want to make it clear," Hertig said, "that they were put on the surgical list by all members of the staff only after it was certain that these women could not avoid hysterectomy. The operation was medically essential. In other words we were not selecting them to put them in that category. They were selected for our studies because they were in that category already. They were having a hysterectomy." In no way was the surgery tantamount to a planned abortion.

But the question hangs in the air. Couldn't the women have been instructed to refrain from marital intercourse and thereby eliminate any possibility of pregnancy at the time of surgery? Hertig vehemently maintained that they were not instructed *to* have intercourse, or *not* to, but only to record it if they did. Were they intelligent enough and informed enough so that they were aware that there was a chance they would be creating a conceptus if they had sex relations? Hertig was confident they were: "I don't think there was any doubt in their minds over this. One of the criteria for their participation in the study was that they had to have had previous children to prove they were fertile. I never discussed it with them. John would." Nonetheless, wouldn't many of those women have considered the result an abortion? "No! How could it be? There was no way in God's world at that time of knowing whether they were pregnant or not. There were literally no tests," Hertig stressed. Diagnosis of pregnancy at the time relied on a woman skipping a menstrual period and subsequent symptoms of breast tenderness and morning sickness.

Even when the first pregnancy lab tests became available, they were not sensitive to hormonal changes in the urine until after the sixth week of pregnancy. Because hormone assay tests today can measure minute changes in hormone levels, if early diagnosis is important, pregnancy can be discerned within a few days. For that reason, it is virtually impossible for the Hertig-Rock experiments to be repeated. Moreover, it is highly unlikely that women could be found, who were in need of a hysterectomy, but who could and would be willing to delay surgery for a few months and spend that time charting their ovulatory cycles, for the sake of an uncertain experiment. In the annals of medicine the work stands alone, a single, brilliant milestone of research in human embryo physiology.

Hertig remembered the first fertilized egg they found. "Well, the lady's name was Mrs. —" he begins the story, obviously enjoying telling it. He speaks with infinite care, scientific accuracy, and in select language. The day in 1938 that the first egg-bearing tissue was brought to him, he was well practiced in the skills needed to bring it to light.

The fresh, still blood-smeared uterus, removed from Mrs. A . . . only minutes earlier, was delivered to him as he waited at his laboratory bench. He followed protocols he'd refined from his Carnegie Institution stint. He placed the specimen, a pear-shaped, thick-walled, muscular organ, a mere three inches long and two inches wide, in a large basin, all the while bathing it in a cleansing saline solution. An assistant held the specimen steady, while Hertig probed for its hidden treasure. Very carefully, he dissected down through the outer walls to the delicate saclike inner lining. Then he incised the sac, bit by bit, until its two sides could be reflected back, laid wide open like the pages of a book. Then he scrupulously scanned the exposed womb lining with a microscope. It had relatively low power, only sixteen times magnification. The field was illuminated with a crudely improvised light, a bull's-eye lamp fitted with a 50-candle-power automobile headlight bulb. Using a needle as a probe, he "dug around" in the tissue to see if a fertilized egg had implanted there. If an egg was not found in the uterus, the fluid used to wash the uterus would be examined to see if it had floated out. A final step was to treat the tissue with Bouin's solution, a cedar oil, that sometimes "brought up" the outline of a missed egg. The solution also shrank and "fixed" the eggs, preserving them. The inside of the Fallopian tubes was similarly inspected. "It was fussy and particular work," Hertig noted.

When, however, late in October 1938, he found the first complete fertilized egg, Hertig says he spotted it instantly. "There was this glistening bead, like a pearl of tapioca. It had a little, tiny red circle around the top of it, which was the internal blood flowing into and through it. The whole diameter was only a single millimeter, one-twenty-fifth of an inch. It was very exciting. There were a lot of hospital people in the laboratory. There was no secrecy about what we were doing. Everyone became very excited because it was the first intact early human ovum implanted in the uterus (womb) that anyone had ever seen.* It was a twelve-day-old conceptus."

With typical old-school loyalty, Hertig and Rock named it the "Harvard egg," nomenclature under which it is forever classified. After examining it, measuring it, and making every possible observation, they "fixed" it with Bouin's solution. That process also clarifies or "clears" tissue, making it semitransparent, much as orange peel is cleared in appearance in marmalade. The specimen was then packaged, as carefully as a "precious biological jewel," which is how Carnegie scientists

---

* Some fertilized human eggs had been found accidentally before this time, in tissue scraped by curettage from the uterus, but they were not intact, nor was their age discernible, and none was as young as the Hertig-Rock collection.

described it. Hertig hand-carried it via airplane to the institution in Baltimore. There, the conceptus (as its successors would be) was photographed, sketched, reexamined, and finally prepared for sectioning so its internal structure could be examined. Only a month or so later, Hertig and Rock found the second egg, an eleven-day-old conceptus. The two became the basis for their first full scientific report of their discoveries.*

Over the next fourteen years, Hertig and Rock collected thirty-four fertilized eggs, gleaned from 211 unknowingly pregnant women. The conceptuses represent the first seventeen days of life.

The Hertig-Rock samples remain the only ones in existence. Their photographs illustrate nearly all medical textbook chapters on embryology. Not each day is accounted for and some of the fertilized eggs were the same age, but Hertig and Rock were able to date the eggs with precision by a combination of measures. The dating of the lining of the womb (which Rock and Dr. Marshall Bartlett had devised) provided one point of reference. The phase of development of the egg itself provided another. For example, the twelve-day-old egg that was found already contained thousands of cells and other internal structures necessary for the fertilized egg's growth and nesting. Finally, of course, age of the conceptus had to dovetail with the woman's record of ovulation and intercourse. In the youngest egg — only thirty-six hours old — the woman had had sexual intercourse only once in the month, just prior to entering the hospital for surgery.

Former Boston Red Sox centerfielder Dominic DiMaggio doesn't know it, but one of the eggs in the famous collection is named for him. It was discovered in October 1946 during the seventh inning of the sixth game of the world series between the Red Sox and the St. Louis Cardinals. At the very moment the egg hove into view beneath Hertig's microscope, DiMaggio hit a long double against the outfield wall. The hit tied up the game, permitting the Sox to win the game, though not the series. Hertig, along with Rock's daughter Rachel, who was working in the lab at the time, was listening to the game. In honor of the two-bagger, and for their private amusement, they christened the egg Dominic. It is Plate #47 in the Carnegie collection.

Hertig and Rock not only supplied the early fertilized eggs, but also

---

* The first egg's discovery had been historically recorded as an abstract in the supplement to the *Anatomy Record* in 1939. The full scientific article appeared in 1941 in *Contributions to Embryology*.

when they had already nested (nidated) in the womb lining, the whole segment was included so others could see the process themselves. They also sent the first samples of virginal eggs, those just emerged, or still bedded within their follicles in the ovary. When possible, Hertig and Rock would also include the segment of the Fallopian tube and/or the empty follicle from which the egg had emerged to demonstrate the anatomical changes occurring as the follicle transformed itself into a miniature progesterone factory.

Thirteen of the eggs were clearly abnormal and twenty-three appeared normal or nearly so. Of the total, only one, the youngest, was found in the Fallopian tube. Seven were still free, not yet attached, in the womb and twenty-six were implanted. Those found to be abnormal in and of themselves, or abnormally implanted, were deemed destined to abort naturally. Often in daily life they pass unnoticed as an abnormally heavy menstrual period before a woman is even aware she had conceived. The collection comprised a new chapter in human embryology, that until then, as Hertig pointed out, "had been a blank, an absolute void. Our specimens filled in a gap of the first days and weeks of human development that had never been seen before."

Their discoveries were of enormous import, often contradicting many of the assumptions of the medical profession about the complex process that results in new life. Rock and Hertig milked the data for every iota of fresh insight that the specimens would yield. They learned some amazing things:

• The presumed twenty-eight-day menstrual cycle was a rarity. Only one of the 211 women whose reproductive organs yielded a conceptus ever had a twenty-eight-day cycle that occurred with regularity. Instead, the cycles varied by as much as seven days in either direction — early or late — from twenty-one to thirty-five days.

• Ovulation did not occur at midcycle as was standardly held. Despite the length of the cycle, ovulation occurred fourteen days (give or take a day or two) before the onset of the next menstrual period. Women relying on rhythm for contraception, therefore, would be seriously misled if they abstained from sex relations strictly at midcycle. Those using rhythm to enhance fertility would be equally misguided.

• The follicle from which the virginal egg emerges, called the corpus luteum or "yellow body" (because it changes from off-white to yellow as it converts into a progesterone-producing gland) has a lifetime of but fourteen days. If the fertilized egg has not begun to attach to the womb lining by that time, the corpus luteum dries up and scars over.

• Virginal eggs that erupt from their follicles right on time (sixteen to fourteen days before the next menstrual period) had a 93.3 percent likelihood of being normal and healthy when fertilized. Only one in thirteen was found likely to be abnormal. Yet, those eggs that erupted even a day later were more than twice as likely to be defective. Examination of the late eggs showed that after fertilization, their rate of growth was slower, somehow stunted.

• Implantation of the fertilized egg in the womb must take place within six days — with very little leeway. Any significant shortening or lengthening of the time is fatal to the budding life.

• Even under the most optimal conditions of timing, receptive tube environment, and healthy egg and sperm, about 15 percent of virginal eggs are consistently lost. They either fail to get into the Fallopian tube because they drop mistakenly into the pelvic cavity or they fail to become fertilized.

• In any one menstrual cycle when all factors are perfect for pregnancy, a woman has a 57.2 percent chance of a good, initial fertilization occurring. Conversely, even under those best-of-all-possible circumstances, there is a 42.8 percent likelihood the cycle will remain sterile.

• If all the eggs that become fertilized however — "good, bad, or indifferent," as Rock and Hertig categorized them — are grouped as 100 percent of the potential pregnancy material, only 71.5 percent are likely to survive the early implantation stage and go on to full term.

• Since some defective as well as sound fertilized eggs begin the implantation process, the life-or-death hurdle for the new conceptus is its capacity to carry out "nesting." The probability of a spontaneous abortion occuring due to inadequate implantation is 28.5 percent.* This observation by Hertig and Rock disclosed that nesting failure accounts for 10 to 15 percent of all infertility in women and so was revealed for the first time as a significant cause of chronic spontaneous abortion.

In 1949 Hertig and Rock won the prestigious American Gynecological Society Award for their painstaking egg work. Hertig fondly recalled that at the ceremonies they were dubbed "the ham and the egg. John was quite an actor you know." With prize in hand, they kissed

* Although only 10 percent of clinically confirmed pregnancies are said to abort, the additional 17 percent are those pregnancies that go unrecognized marked only by a delayed, heavy menstrual period. The conceptus is passed as part of the menstrual cellular debris without the woman ever knowing she was pregnant.

one another, an uncommon gesture of their affection and one rarely expressed between American men, especially scientists. "I loved him and he loved me and we did our work. It's as simple as that. We all adored him. He was an elite kind of scientist, well educated — really educated. He had enormous respect for the patients. John is a good example of the cultured individual who was devoted to his work and his patients. We were very committed, pretty much with our lives. It wasn't . . . the interest wasn't in making money. It was knowledge we were after." Rock felt the same way: "That's a piece of work I'm really proud of. It was a major contribution to the knowledge of human reproduction." Though Hertig continued the egg hunt after 1953, by which time he'd taken over the pathology department at HMS and largely moved his base of operation to the more conveniently located Boston Lying-In Hospital, only one more fertilized egg was ever turned up. Amazingly, while the Hertig-Rock collection of fertilized eggs was regarded as one of the pinnacles of research among embryologists, the public knew next to nothing about it. A brief account of the first two eggs was reported in the Boston press in April 1939 — when Hertig described the work before a professional society. The only major news story appeared in September 1966, disseminated by the Associated Press and based on a report about the full collection by Hertig at the annual meeting in Washington, D.C., of the American Society of Clinical Pathologists. The news versions made no mention of John Rock.

Stylistically, Hertig and Rock had much in common, though they were opposite physically. Both men were gregarious and very sociable. Both savored literary language, precisely used, and they liked a good time, good company, good food, good wine, and good conversation. Both had an educated ear for classical music. Nothing interfered with Hertig's attendance of the Boston Symphony Orchestra in season. Both were a touch vain about their clothing, and dressed very distinctively. But Hertig did not have as great a flair for showmanship as Rock, he readily admitted. With open admiration he recalled a gynecological meeting in Hot Springs, Arkansas, when Rock came into the convention room near the end of the program. Someone in the audience asked Rock to discuss a very technical point that had been raised in one of the papers presented. Rock tried to fob the question to Hertig, who handed it right back to Rock. "John went up to the podium and gave an absolutely remarkable discourse on the subject, never having heard the paper at all," Hertig marveled. They were together during some very dark moments, too. Hertig was with Rock at another scientific meeting in West Point, New York, in 1959 when Rock received word his wife had cancer of the colon. "He was a good surgeon and he knew what the diagnosis meant. The news hit him hard, very hard. He never really got over it."

No one knew better than Hertig the thoroughness of their joint research or what a stickler for accuracy and clarity Rock was. Hertig also knew the force and vitality given the work by Rock's personality. "In the first place, he was fun to work with. He was always excited about what he was doing and that kind of animation was infectious for all of us. The whole problem with fertility and infertility was a big thing and we had a sense that what we were doing was really important. I thought it was great fun to work under him. He was enthusiastic and stimulating and outgoing. He had true charisma." When Rock reached mandatory retirement age in 1956, it was Hertig who "got his emeritus" for him. "I was a friend of George Packer Berry, who was the dean then of Harvard Medical School. And besides, Rock deserved it. He'd only been a clinical professor and so it was exceptional that he was designated emeritus. John had a great deal of modesty. He didn't toot his own horn." Hertig believed that "Harvard medical politics" had a good deal to do with Rock's never rising to become chief at the Free Hospital. Others felt that Rock's Catholicism was the biggest stumbling block. Hertig deservedly rose to chairman of the department of pathology and held the named chair, the Shattuck Professor of Pathological Anatomy at Harvard Medical School, until his retirement in 1970. Since then, he has continued as chairman of the division of pathobiology at the Harvard-affiliated New England Regional Primate Research Center in Southborough, Massachusetts.

At the peak of their collaborative research, however, Hertig and Rock, in producing the first material evidence of the earliest stages of human life, set in motion very far-reaching first steps. They put in place the underpinnings for the latter-day application of test-tube conception. The spectacular payoff did not come for forty-one years, until 1979 with the birth of "Baby Louise" Brown in England, the first child to be conceived outside her mother's womb — literally in a watch glass* — and then implanted within her mother to gestate and be born naturally. Among other important information gleaned from the early-stage fertilized eggs, Rock and Hertig sorted out characteristics by

---

* Its name refers to the thick bottom, a disc similar to the face of a watch. These, not test-tubes are used for so-called test-tube conception.

which the eggs could be judged biologically, "good, bad or indifferent." Thus, the Hertig-Rock collection gave the first solid basis upon which selection of "good" eggs — those suitable for test-tube conception and implantation — can be made from their microscopic appearance.

"I have no illusions about how I, or any of us for that matter, fits into the whole scheme of things," Hertig wrote, summing up his career. "We are all dwarfs standing on the shoulders of giants, the greater to increase our view. When one stands back and reviews one's scientific life, it is as though one were looking at a grand picture puzzle. One can say, 'See that little piece? I put it in!' We all profit from our teachers. I have had some great ones in my time from several scientific disciplines. I have been fortunate in having had the fruitful collaboration with Dr. John Rock."

Hertig remained convinced that there was little correlation between quality of work and the fanciness of laboratory surroundings. "What we still need is a few more high-powered workers with lower-powered tools," he once said. Rock had just such a worker in the redoubtable Miriam Menkin. While Hertig and Rock were looking for fertilized eggs, Rock and Miriam undertook no less a challenge than to attempt the first human conception in a test tube.

5

TEST-TUBE FERTILIZATION

JOHN ROCK met Miriam Menkin for the first time early in March 1938. She'd heard of a job opening in his laboratory and had come for an interview. All the way over, in her self-deprecating way, she'd rehearsed in her mind how she would tell him about the graduate work and research she'd done at Harvard and with Gregory Pincus, "all that stuff," in the hope it would persuade him to hire her. A week earlier she'd sent a letter outlining her educational and scientific credentials. Having read the letter, Rock didn't bother to inquire about any of it. He asked her only three questions.

"Do you drink?" She answered no.

"Then he asked, as though it were the most ordinary sort of inquiry, 'How would you like to fertilize an egg?' " She said with equal equanimity, she would.

All he wanted to know after that was how soon she could start. She told him the next day. From that casual beginning would come medical history.

Miriam Menkin is absolutely one of a kind: a singular sort of unsung heroine in the center of a drama in which figures and forces intertwine, moving and shaping what was destined to be an epochal moment in scientific research. Though her personal life was cruel, bitter, disheartening, and disruptive, she bore it all willingly. She managed against a veritable onslaught of obstacles to hold on to the one thing she cherished above all else — the chance to work with Rock. "I wouldn't change places with anyone in the world. The privilege of being in his company and the chance to work on such a monumental project — fertilization *in vitro* [in glass] — was the greatest thing in the world," she believes to this day. The most ardent feminist of today would be hard put to endure what Miriam Menkin went through in order to remain an active scientist. It is no exaggeration that her sacrifices rival those of Madame Curie.

The wife of Valy Menkin, a young Harvard medical student, Miriam had come to Boston in 1924 as his bride. Uncommonly beautiful, delicately boned, and with large, wide-set eyes, she was finely intelligent, though she often seemed a bit distracted. She was an exceedingly well trained biologist for her time. Born in a tiny village outside Riga, Latvia, in 1901, she had come to the United States as a two-year-old, when her father, Dr. Gedide Abraham Friedman, immigrated to this country. An older brother, her parents' only son, died in early childhood. Miriam became a surrogate son to her father, who vested in her his dreams of having a child follow him into medicine. Her pianist mother, Ida, wanted Miriam to be a musician. Her life became a torment of conflicting expectations: her parents', her husband's, her own; and eventually, her children's.

She was awarded her Bachelor of Arts degree in science, specifically embryology and histology, from Cornell University in 1922, as a pre-med major. She was a dedicated student earning high honors even though she was debilitated by extremely heavy menstrual periods caused by endometriosis.* She took her master's degree from Columbia University in zoology with special emphasis on the then still new science of genetics. Her life at home in New York City was gracious and comfortable, one of abundant money, household help, and social position. "I never learned to cook or sew or do anything useful," she recalled self-demeaningly.

In marrying Valy Menkin, she assumed financial responsibility for supporting both of them and helped pay his way through medical school.† Working in one misbegotten laboratory job after another, she

---

* Abnormal bleeding from segments of the endometrium, the tissue that appropriately lines the womb but is misplaced elsewhere in the pelvis. Ironically, the pill is now the treatment of choice for the condition.

† In time he achieved distinction with his work on the understanding of immunological shock; particularly the mechanisms of inflammatory chain reaction that occurs when the human system is traumatized by severe injury, infection, or burns.

clung to the vain hope that she, too, would one day become an M.D., or get her doctorate degree in biology. Twice, on the free-of-charge auditing basis, she completed the requirements for a Ph.D. degree at Harvard, but never had enough money to pay the course fee whereby the degree could be awarded her. She was fluent in French and German as well as English and had a passing acquaintance with Russian, her parents' and husband's native tongue. To help her husband prepare his school papers, she also mastered shorthand and typing. After his graduation, she assisted him occasionally on projects at Harvard Medical School where he worked as a research pathologist.

One day, while she was so employed, Gregory Pincus came in and offered her a job. He was trying to extract two hormones from the pituitary gland in the brain, hormones that act as override regulators of the male and female reproductive cycle. The offer was to drastically alter the course of her life. One of the hormones Pincus was interested in is called follicle stimulating hormone (FSH). It causes ovarian follicles to step up their production of the female sex hormone estrogen and thereby ripen an egg for ovulation. The other hormone was luteinizing hormone (LH), which transforms the emptied follicle after ovulation into the corpus luteum, the miniature gland that produces the other female sex hormone, progesterone. Progesterone, the classic hormone of pregnancy, readies the womb to receive and support a fertilized egg, should conception occur. The job that Pincus offered Miriam paid fifty dollars a month.

Though married twelve years, Miriam and Valy were childless and the marriage was on the verge of collapse. She put away the fifty-dollar stipends so that she could afford to leave him. In Pincus's lab she succeeded in isolating some FSH and LH from a preparation of sheep pituitary-gland extract. She pipetted off some of the superfluous fluid and must have swallowed some. Until then, she had not been able to get pregnant because she didn't ovulate. "The FSH evidently stimulated my system to ovulate because I conceived Gabriel [her son] at that very time," she maintains.* The pregnancy ended any hope of her separating from her husband. "I was pregnant. I couldn't leave him then." Typically, she was so preoccupied with her work she didn't notice that she was skipping periods — the classic sign of pregnancy — for five

---

* If her assumption is correct, she would be the first woman in history to ovulate and conceive as a direct result of taking FSH — a substance later used for that very purpose in women who were sterile because they were anovulatory.

months! When she told her obstetrician that she thought it was the FSH that had overcome her previous infertility and suggested other women might try it, he said such a trial would have to be carried out by an expert, like John Rock. That was the first time she had heard John Rock's name.

Gabriel was born in October 1936 and Miriam heard no more of Rock for two years. Determined to work despite her motherhood and, worse, a stone wall of resistance against her as a married woman, she also was stymied by more subtle but equally injurious anti-Semitism. On two occasions after being accepted for jobs, the offer was withdrawn when it was learned she was Jewish. Once, while on a tour of a Boston hospital, the guide paused to call attention to an unexpected point of interest. Indicating the presence of a man whom Miriam recognized as a leading authority on X-rays, the guide exclaimed, "and that's a *Jew!*" After many frustrations, Miriam took a qualifying exam for a Civil Service appointment as a laboratory technician and came out first on the list for the entire state. Finally, she was hired to work in the state biological laboratories in Jamaica Plain, where a new test for syphilis was being evaluated. It was a frightful job. She had to climb ladders to reach cages containing "these tremendous dogs that looked like horses to me or drag down overgrown rabbits. Half of all the animals had syphilis. My job was to inject them with biologicals for the study. I wanted to quit every day but I couldn't because every time a rabbit bit you, you had to go take a Wassermann test to make sure you hadn't contracted syphilis. Finally I just beat it, never went back and never put in for my pay — eighty dollars." At this time, she again heard of Rock and a job opening in his laboratory, and the fateful interview took place.

With Miriam's arrival, Rock really launched the "egg hunt." She was vital to the project. Rock wanted two types of eggs: fertilized eggs for the project with Hertig; and unfertilized eggs for attempts at test-tube conception. The only way to get them was from women undergoing hysterectomies. But the right patients had to be found, and Miriam was the perfect intermediary.

It worked this way. First Miriam checked the list of all clinic patients assigned for surgery. The "candidates," as they were called, had to meet certain criteria. They had to be married, under forty-five years old, and already have at least two children — some had fourteen — to prove they were fertile. Their diagnosis had to be suitable: serious enough to warrant a hysterectomy but not so diseased that they could no longer ovulate or conceive. Miriam would select the most promising among them, those who also seemed intelligent and dependable. Rock would double-check to make sure all the conditions were met. Then Miriam would contact the women, explain the research, and ask if they were willing to participate. From those who agreed, she took a menstrual history and arranged for them to come in so Rock could give them a thorough gynecologic examination. After that, she taught them how to keep a calendar chart of their reproductive cycle. They were to take their temperature each morning before arising, and particularly, note the midcycle dip and rise of body temperature which signifies ovulation. At that time of the month, the Catholic women were taught how to practice "rhythm" — an appropriate period of sexual abstinence; and non-Catholics advised to use whatever form of contraception was acceptable to them. The women followed this routine for six monthly cycles until the month prior to their surgery. Such instruction in birth control was, of course, illegal in Massachusetts.

At this point Rock and Hertig's version of the instructions given the women differs somewhat from Miriam's. But it was she, not they, who was dealing directly with the "candidates." Rock and Hertig hold that the women were advised in that final month to continue their normal pattern of sexual intercourse — but this time without using any precautions to prevent conception. The women were asked to keep a record of the dates of any intercourse, and that was all. Miriam says there was a little more than that to it. Miriam would point out to the candidates "these other women sitting on the bench in the infertility clinic. They are women who would like to have a baby, who can't. We want to find out more about how to help them by finding out more about the early stages of a baby." She would reassure the women that "even if you have intercourse you won't have a baby because you have to have the operation anyway." She would hint at least that it would be *useful* to the research if they had intercourse during the final fertile period. "After all," she rationalized, "the practical fact of it was that there wasn't much point in going to all the trouble of preparing the women for the study, if none were going to at least give their eggs a chance to be exposed to their husband's sperm. There was a crude pregnancy test at the time but it couldn't work until a woman was six to eight weeks pregnant. Neither we nor they could know whether they were pregnant at the time of surgery."

Week after week, the "candidates" would bring in their reproductive cycle charts and Miriam would try to ascertain when they were most likely to ovulate. Rock would ask her to see if she could calculate the timing to try for "an embryo on day fifteen, sixteen, or seventeen of the menstrual cycle. I was a nervous wreck. I guess most anyone would be. What if they had a cold or something when they came to the hospital for surgery and therefore couldn't be operated on. Then, they could miss a period and know they were pregnant." Only once was a "mistake" made. One woman just didn't disclose that her period was overdue. For her, that slip amounted to going forward consciously with an abortion. Rock, however, was unaware of it when he performed the hysterectomy. Proof that she, indeed, was pregnant came when her womb was found to contain a seventeen-day conceptus, the oldest in the collection.

For their test-tube conception research, Rock and Miriam at first tried to dovetail surgery precisely with the patient's anticipated day of ovulation. Soon, however, they learned that the patient only had to be close to ovulation time. They could do as well by gathering nearly ripe eggs from the excised ovaries. The nearly ripe eggs could be brought to full maturity by incubating them in the donor's blood serum for a day or two. After that, when a "candidate's" ovulation time coincided with a Tuesday, she was scheduled for surgery on that day — Rock's regular day in surgery for clinic patients. The maneuver put the test-tube conception study on a weekly routine.

One of the strangest rituals in medical history then began. Every Tuesday morning Miriam would wait, like a sentry on guard, outside the operating room on the ground floor of the Parkway wing of the Free Hospital. In her hands she carried a jar of sterile solution. Her vigil began at eight o'clock, the time surgery began. Sometimes she would have collected the specimens — wedges or complete ovaries, Fallopian tubes, and wombs — by nine-thirty. More often, however, she would still be standing there at midafternoon. There were no phones connecting the operating room to the laboratory which would have made it possible for her simply to respond to a summons at the right moment. But it was essential that she get the eggs immediately, while they were still alive and before they would begin to disintegrate. For six years, she kept watch by the OR door each Tuesday, collecting the tissue containing the precious eggs.

She would then hurry to Rock's small laboratories on the third floor. There she delicately made a fine incision in the Fallopian tube, hold it over a watch glass (a small, round laboratory dish with shallow sides and open at the top) and, using Locke's solution, flush the contents into the dish. If an egg were in the tube, she would use a needle as a makeshift miniature scalpel and painstakingly clean away any tubal cells that might be stuck to it. With ovaries, or segments of them, the procedure was slightly different. Since ovaries are composed of little sacs that are partially transparent and filled with fluid covered over by a membrane, she would divide the ovary into wedges. Then, selecting the largest sacs (follicles) that looked as though they might contain ripe or nearly ripe eggs, she would puncture the surface membrane and let the contents drain into a watch glass.

Whatever the source, the eggs were gently washed three times by pipetting Locke's solution over them. The eggs next were transferred into a fat-bottomed, narrow-necked Carrel flask, containing three cubic centimeters of blood from the patient. Miriam pointed out that "no one knew what the best culture medium for them was, but I just thought that the simplest thing was what was nearest to the egg. That was the woman who supplied it, so I thought her blood was best." Sometimes in pipetting the eggs from the watch glass to the flask, she'd lose the egg, finding it days later stuck in the pipette. Actually the pipettes used were pipulettes, an extremely finely calibrated hollow glass tube.

In the lab her next move was to take the egg, now nestling in its donor's blood, and incubate it at body temperature (37.5 degrees Celsius) for twenty-four hours. During that time, the ripening egg would cast off the extra set of chromosomes it carried during its immature phase of development. (A mature egg has only twenty-three chromosomes to pair with twenty-three from the sperm, thus creating the forty-six-chromosome normal complement of genetic material in each human cell, one half derived from each parent.) Presence of a "polar body," the cast-off, excess twenty-three chromosomes, was evidence the egg had properly ripened and was ready for fertilization.

The day-long incubation period conveniently made time for the most anonymous player in the drama to be brought in: one of the coterie of sperm donors, who were on call. That task was delicately left to Rock, who had a roster of young interns available on short notice. They were particularly amenable to his requests. Not only did he pay a small fee, but he also made the process of donation as palatable as possible. In the private cubicle where donors would masturbate and ejaculate the semen samples into a sterile container, Rock hung large posters of voluptuous nudes which he'd picked up in Sweden to help "inspire the young men to action."

The samples of sticky semen, each containing 300 million or so sperm, would be given to Miriam. She would spin off (centrifuge) the liquid, leaving the sperm to settle to the bottom of a test tube. As with the egg, the sperm also had to be washed three times in Locke's solution — not to clean them, but to activate them. To be able to fertilize an egg, sperm must pass through a preparatory phase, called capacitation, in which a latent enzyme (hyaluronidase) is released. In the human system, capacitation takes place in the womb or Fallopian tube, which supplies secretions that uncap the sperm head. Thence, when an activated sperm encounters an egg, the sperm is able to release an enzyme that breaks down a cementlike substance that seals the outer layer of the egg. The seal must be broken for the sperm to penetrate the egg wall.

From his laboratory, at that time at Clark University in Worcester, Gregory Pincus played a tangential role in the Rock-Menkin attempts at test-tube conception. The incubation technique employed by Miriam was a modification of a method Pincus had originated at Harvard when he was first attempting to ripen rabbit eggs. She occasionally telephoned him to test out ideas or for reassurance. Later, it was Pincus's protégé, Min-Chueh Chang, who unraveled the mystery of sperm capacitation, showing that the substance that triggers sperm capacitation is albumen, an essential protein commonly found in blood, milk, and egg white. Since small amounts of albumen are present in Locke's solution, in which Miriam bathed the sperm, she unwittingly succeeded in activating the sperm, although she had no idea what the ignition factor was at the time.

Seated at her lab bench, Miriam next would take the egg out of the incubator. "It would still be in the one-cell stage, of course. Sometimes I could see the vague outline of the first polar body. It looked like a small, dark shadow off to one side within the egg. I would move the egg into a watch glass, again in Locke's solution, and add the sperm. The sperm could not be added to the blood serum containing the egg, because blood clumps sperm together, killing them. I found that out after a long time of doing it wrong." Then she would sit with the watch glass in focus under a microscope and watch the sperm wriggle and, then, mass around the egg, varying the time from fifteen minutes to half an hour.

After the attempt at mating in the watch glass, she would once more bathe the egg and sperm in Locke's solution and then transfer them to a flask. This time the flask contained blood from a post-menopausal woman, so chosen because Miriam felt it would be more constant, and not vary in its hormonal content. Again the flask would return to the incubator for forty-eight hours, now hopefully containing "conceived" human life. Week after week for six years, she obtained the eggs on Tuesday, added the sperm on Wednesday, went home and "prayed all day Thursday." Late on Friday, some forty-six to forty-eight hours later, each week she took out the little flask again and placed it under a microscope. The incubator-warmed flask would cause steam to form on the cold microscope lens. She would hold a lighted match near the field of the microscope to clear away the blurring steam, and look to see if the precious quarry they sought were there . . . a fertilized human egg. It always was discouragingly the same as it had been to begin with . . . a still virginal egg. At first Miriam repeated the process one egg at a time. Later, she would extract "a whole bunch of eggs" and expose them to sperm simultaneously. She tried it with nearly a thousand eggs culled from hundreds of women. Still nothing happened.

Then, in 1935, Miriam was pregnant again. Her home life had become a shambles, beset with domestic problems. Her husband lost his Harvard position. Her mother, suffering a nervous breakdown, lived nearby and was a constant worry. Miriam's devotion to the lab at all hours of the day and night infuriated her husband. There were terrible fights, with everyone shouting. It was just "a crazy house," Miriam said. So far as her work was concerned, she ignored her condition and made little of the demands that pulled her in every direction. "Getting a fertilized egg" was what mattered most. On those occasions when eggs were obtained late in the day, she would return to the laboratory at two and three o'clock in the morning the following day to fertilize them on schedule; even when she was pregnant. She still vividly remembers how her back ached from bending over the microscope for long stretches at a time. "It's a good thing there weren't many muggers in those days," she noted, "because we lived in a lonely section of Brookline about three blocks away from the hospital. It was pretty eerie when I'd have to dash over there in the middle of the night to treat the eggs."

She worked until four in the afternoon the Saturday before the Monday when Lucy was born — a week late — in June 1943. Rock would throw up his hands in mock horror at the sight of her and say, "Are you still here!" Because she was on the regular payroll at the time, she was entitled to two weeks' paid vacation. They were the first and last she would ever have. She spent them in the hospital having Lucy, returning to the lab seventeen days after the delivery. Rock was startled and more than a little concerned to find her back. "He was very mad at me, especially when he found I had climbed the hill to the hospital. He personally ordered cab service for me to and from work for several weeks after that." Rock also wrote her a "beautiful letter, very complimentary," which she forwarded to her father. Rock said that in caring for thousands of pregnant women, he'd never seen another woman who had gone through pregnancy and childbirth with the fortitude Miriam showed.

Just before Lucy was born, however, Miriam, while attempting to fertilize some eggs, had intermixed eggs from the ovaries of two different women. "I was tired," she says, "and I guess I was short a few — I tried to do a dozen at a time — and so I took a batch of eggs from two different patients. I didn't know which was which. I don't know whether that made some difference in the mix, but what was produced was really a monster. It was the weirdest looking thing and grew to have about fifteen cells." It, of course, was the first test-tube human fertilization, but was never reported. Miriam "fixed" it with preservative, however, and saved it. "Just at that point Lucy was born, so I couldn't do anything about it." Lucy's arrival, however, did not distract her from probing further into the strange cluster of cells. When Lucy was six weeks old, Miriam took the specimen and made the forty-mile trip by bus to Worcester to show it to Pincus. "He looked at it and was very impressed. It was a weird-looking thing and he saw that it was definitely abnormal. Of course, I was thrilled. It was the first time I'd gotten anything that was more than one cell — the naked egg, itself. So I had done something different when I got that one, but I didn't know what it was. I think, now, I must have kept the egg and sperm together longer that night because I was so tired." She kept on trying.

The history-making moment came on Friday, February 6, 1944. The previous Tuesday, Miriam gathered eggs from ovarian tissue taken from a thirty-eight-year-old married woman, who'd had four children. She'd been admitted for a hysterectomy because she suffered long, hard pregnancies and labors that had lacerated and eroded the cervix (neck of the womb) and so overstretched the muscles that support the womb they lost all their elasticity. The womb had prolapsed down through the weakened cervix, protruding into the vaginal canal. The woman's cycles had been followed for four months, pre-operatively. When the hysterectomy was performed, the womb was removed and the Fallopian tube and ovary on the right side — leaving the left intact, as was often done then, to maintain a source of estrogen production. Because she had a short cycle, the operation was performed on the tenth day of the woman's menstrual cycle. Rock had learned that ovulation was not so much midcycle as fourteen days preceding the next menstrual period. At surgery, he found he was correct. All the signs that ovulation was imminent were present. The woman never knew it, but she was to become the mother-in-absentia of the first conception in a test tube.

Miriam flushed out a likely-looking egg about an hour after the ovary was removed. She took it through the ordered steps, washed it, incubated it, and went home. She was up the whole night with Lucy, who at eight months of age was cutting her first tooth. The next morning, Wednesday, Miriam added sperm to the incubated and, thus, mature egg, the way she'd done so many hundreds of times before. "I must have dozed off," she says. She left the watch glass containing the egg and sperm on the dissecting microscope stage for an hour — far longer than ever before. "What happened, I think, was that I was so exhausted that I became mesmerized as I sat there and watched the sperm wriggle and mass around the egg. Those sperm, they're so active that they actually twirl the egg around. Nothing I've ever seen is really as thrilling as that . . . to sit and watch and think that from this comes a baby. So I sat there and watched this beautiful thing, that to me is the most wonderful sight in the world. Even if I had Liz Taylor's diamonds, I wouldn't think they were as glamorous as seeing this egg and the spermatozoa whirling it round and round. Not many people have seen it. At that time nobody else in the world had seen human egg and sperm attempting to unite, but Dr. Rock and me. I must have grown groggy watching it and nodded off. Then, I sort of came to and found it was a much longer length of time than the fifteen minutes to half an hour that I'd used before."

The sperm showed great activity, she noticed. They could clearly be seen to travel through the debris around the egg. Many could be seen in active motion around the zona pellucida (the surface tissue) that encloses the genetic material inside.

She removed the sperm-swarmed egg, rebathed it in Locke's solution, and reimmersed it in blood; this time the serum from a fifty-one-year-old menopausal woman. "As the egg was pipetted back into the Carrel flask," she vividly recalled, "the loose formation of degenerated tissue cells that were attached to it suddenly dropped off. It appeared as a single round cell with a fuzzy border." She set the specimen back in the incubator and left it there for the standard two days. In this case, exactly forty-seven hours.

"I never did anything on Thursday. I just stayed home and prayed, as usual. Friday I went in to the lab and went to the incubator and took the specimen out. I couldn't see anything different with my naked eye, so I set it to one side. About ten or eleven in the morning I put the little flask under my dissecting microscope, lit a match to clear away the steam, and took a look. I had always wondered, after six years of trying, what I would say or do if suppose it did happen . . . if I really saw a two-cell egg. Well, I found out.

"When I saw it, I began to scream. A lady in the next room (actually Mrs. Snedeker in charge of the Rhythm Clinic) said she was doing some paperwork and heard me say, sounding hysterical, 'Oh my heavens, I should have done those eye exercises.' " Miriam thought she was seeing double. A few months before an eye doctor had found a muscle defect in her eyes and prescribed eye exercises. He'd warned her that if she didn't do them, she would "wake up one morning and find that she was seeing double." She could never bother with them, so her first reaction to the sight of the fertilized egg was that her eyesight indeed had failed. "Then, I realized what it was, that it was real, a genuine fertilized egg. I nearly dropped dead. Dr. Rock wasn't around. He was at the Phillips House [Mass. General Hospital] delivering a baby.

"I was so excited and so frightened I was shaking like a leaf. I took the elevator down one flight to Dr. Hertig's office. I didn't dare walk down the stairs. He was at his microscope, but he was about to leave and was annoyed at first that I was delaying him. Then, he saw the state I was in. He said I was trembling as though I were on the verge of a stroke. I just stood there. He said I was very pale. I could barely speak. Finally, I said, 'Dr. Hertig, would you come upstairs and see what I just saw.' He did, and saw the same thing and started calling everybody in the hospital. They all came over. The laboratory was full of people. And there I was sitting there in their midst with this beautiful two-celled egg.

"I felt like — who was the first man to look at the Pacific — Balboa?" Miriam said. "You see, I really was nobody. If you don't get a doctorate in this kind of field [embryology], you always work under other people. You're in a different category. You may want to do independent work, but you're not allowed to. But there it was . . . the first fertilized egg . . . what no one had ever done before." It justified all the hardships she had endured.

A great discussion ensued over how best to preserve the wondrous egg. Miriam wanted to do it the quick, easy way. But Hertig and others opted for a safer process for preserving the precious find, but one that was less familiar, extremely intricate, and took several hours. Pencil sketches were immediately made of the conceptus and then Miriam settled down to carry out the fussy preservation as she was instructed. In the process she lost the egg. By the time Rock got to the lab it was gone. Over the weekend, she returned to the lab repeatedly, searching frantically for it. By Monday, all hope of finding it — stuck to the edge of a dish or caught in a pipette — was lost. Miriam was disconsolate over what Rock would think of her. "He came in all full of smiles," she recalled, "and said, 'Well, let's have a look at it.' I had to tell him it was lost." With typical equanimity, he just shrugged, "his expression never changes, you know, and he said, 'That's understandable. After all, it was just a little thing.' " Eventually, they came to think of it as the first miscarriage *in vitro*.

They started again. From then on, however, Miriam exposed the harvested eggs to the longer fertilization time, a full hour, in the watch glass with sperm. Within a few months, she repeated the accomplishment — three times. Twice more she coaxed an egg and sperm to mate in the small watch glass and to go through at least one stage of cell division. With a third egg, she brought it through two stages of division. These times, she held on to the tiny conceptuses and Hertig photographed them, immediately. Then, Miriam preserved them, each time transferring the tiny bits of human protoplasm to a drop of blood plasma, and then fixing them in Bouin's solution, drying them by the warmth of a lamp, and nestling them in a celluloid-paraffin bed.

One of the specimens was cut open and sectioned (microscopically sliced like a loaf of bread) for further examination. The study revealed that the egg and sperm, indeed, had united to start the journey by which every human travels into life. Not only was the conceptus characterized by changes of inner cell division, certain dark shadows were suggestive of a sperm head, one of which appeared just inside the cell body of the conceptus. The test-tube embryos were so precious that they, too, were hand-carried by Hertig to the Carnegie Institution in Maryland, where they remain preserved in the Department of Embryology. Their photographs, also, illustrate many textbooks on embryology.

In contrast to the absence of public attention paid the Hertig-Rock early egg collection, the first report of the test-tube fertilization hit the newsstands on August 4, 1944. The scientific report was carried in *Science* magazine. Popular versions moved on the Associated Press national news wire under the by-line of the AP's distinguished science writer Howard Blakeslee.* As the stories reached the public and the science community, Rock lay in a hospital bed in the Phillips House at the MGH, beginning to recover from a major heart attack, the first of the six to strike him over the next thirty years. Lying there, he at least took satisfaction that the AP story was reasonably accurate and put the findings in perspective:

> The first artificial fertilization of human ova, or eggs, in a glass test tube, entirely outside the bodies of the mothers and fathers, was announced today in the journal *Science*.
>
> Although this is technically the first step in test tube babies, which for years have been rumored in laboratories, the experiments indicate absolutely no way to produce babies artificially.
>
> They are a medical study of the very first steps of human conception. Two of these human eggs developed into two cells each, and a third developed further into three cells.
>
> These early steps are impossible to observe in life. The technique makes them visible for the first time. Everything in this study was done under the eye of a microscope with photographic attachments which made a permanent record.
>
> One special purpose of the study was to get information on the rather baffling problem of human sterility. . . .

In the news report Blakeslee also observed:

> After fertilization the first cleavage is the first step in development of a living body. It is the beginning of formation of the billions of tissue cells which finally form a complete individual. Along with the increase in tissue cells goes the appearance from time to time of many different kinds of tissue cells, which ultimately form the widely varied tissues and structures of the human body.

Science News Service pointed out in its news copy that "the experiments have enabled scientists to observe for the first time, some of the events of the first few hours of human prenatal existence, and may

* Except in the *New York Times*, which dropped his name from the story.

eventually open the way for better understanding of still-obscure points in embryology."

As background, Science News Service noted that "artificially controlled manipulation of animal development from eggs began a half-century or so ago when zoologists were able to produce fatherless worms, sea urchins and even frogs by stimulating infertilized eggs with chemicals, needle scratches and electric current. More recently, Dr. Gregory Pincus now at Clark University, was able to remove unfertilized eggs of living rabbits and start development by similar procedures. . . . Dr. Rock and Miss [sic] Menkin state that they received assistance from Dr. Pincus in their present series of experiments."

The news stories catapulted Rock to instant fame. While it is true that over time fame is fleeting, nonetheless, as the news reports reverberated around the world, they were enough to begin to attract an untoward reaction at Harvard that would cost Rock dearly in later years. But the immediate effect of the news coverage was to prompt hundreds of people to write to him. Mail poured in from all over the country. Some inquiries came from women who had functioning ovaries and wombs, but lacked the vital connecting link, Fallopian tubes (as did Baby Louise's mother). They wanted Rock to take their "good eggs" and fertilize them in his laboratory and replace them inside their womb. One letter came from a self-made corporation head who wanted Rock and Miriam to find a woman with good eggs to act as a natural incubator for his exceptionally worthy sperm. His own wife had "something the matter" with her. Other mail came in, too, from outraged readers, most of them Catholics, who accused Rock and Miriam of "playing God," committing abortion, and of being scientific fiends. Another demanded that they make sure they would be "able to raise and educate properly" any children who would come out of such experiments.

By a quirk of chance, Rock was spared a confrontation with the cardinal who had officiated at his marriage. William Cardinal O'Connell, the first cardinal ever appointed for New England, died on April 14, four months before the news reports of the conception in a test tube hit the newsstands. Interestingly, no *formal* move was ever made against Rock by the Catholic Church, by the watchdog Massachusetts legislature, or even by the ever-vigilant righteous in a repressive, Puritan-minded state. Nineteen forty-four, however, was a very touchy year for such experiments to be announced. A referendum question seeking to end the state's ban on birth control was once again on the ballot. As always, the politics surrounding the referendum question were bitter, pitting Catholic Democrats and Protestant Republicans against one another in an intense confrontation. As with abortion in 1981, birth control was denounced from the altar by Catholic priests, acting under instructions from the new head of the archdiocese, Archbishop Richard Cushing. Behind the scenes, Harvard antagonists of Rock's are said to have exerted their influence to make sure that any further experiments by him in the same vein were squashed, or at least subverted.

"The termination of a pregnancy surgically, even though you couldn't diagnose the pregnancy at the time, put the work in a border area ethically, a gray zone," Dr. Celso-Ramon Garcia pointed out. (Later he was a co-investigator with Rock on the pill.) While there was no way Rock could be accused of being an abortionist, yet, because there was a probability factor of pregnancy, there was that threat. That threat became very real when the results of their experiments were published. Although Rock was very clear in his mind of the rightness of what they had done, he had no taste for being a martyr. He and Miriam had reached a very important level of discovery. He didn't abandon the work but it wasn't worth pressing his luck to expand it. There was no denying the subject was supersensitive, and not only with Catholics. No money was made available to continue the test-tube conception research in any form.

Miriam and Rock, however, planned to go on quietly on their own. It was not to be. Life has short-changed Miriam Menkin in myriad ways, but probably most cruelly at that moment. Her husband lost his job at the Fearing Laboratory at the Free Hospital. He found a new appointment at Duke University in North Carolina. His job change meant she and the children would have to move there with him. Rock pleaded with Harvard Medical School dean George Packer Berry to give Valy another position, if only out of consideration of the important work that Rock, Hertig, and Miriam had under way collecting fertilized eggs. Berry wouldn't do it. The test-tube-conception work was stalemated. Continuance of such laboratory trifling with human life would have amounted to a direct affront to the Catholic hierarchy, particularly in Boston, which could have been difficult for Harvard. In any case, Valy Menkin found no reprieve and the whole family had to move on. Miriam was crushed. Rock tried to resume the work by training another assistant, but it never got off the ground again.

If family life was turbulent in Massachusetts for the Menkins, it was tumultuous at Duke. They never really settled into a home, moving instead from hotel to hotel. Within two years Valy moved on to a post in the pathology department at Temple University in Philadelphia. Miriam, meanwhile, still had to prepare substantial sections of the full report on test-tube fertilization. To do it she needed a medical library where she could research historic precedents for the work. The nearest was in the city several miles from their North Philadelphia home. The faithful but domineering housekeeper Agnes had moved along with the family, but she would only allow Miriam to be away from the house for three hours during the morning. To get to the library, Miriam traveled by bus and subway for an hour and one-quarter each way. That left her half an hour in the library. A stickler for details and for giving credit where it was due, she ferreted out every possible previous animal study related to test-tube conception. (Rock, though admiring, would often complain that she went all the way back to Egyptian papyri for sources.) On her backbreaking travel schedule, it took three years to finish her contribution to the report. When it was published as an "original communication" in the *Journal of Obstetrics and Gynecology* in 1948, she listed twenty-two references, dating back to 1880 and included works in Russian, German, and French as well as English. Rock, generously, listed her name first as co-author. Publication of the full report brought Miriam additional recognition. In April 1948 she was invited to discuss the test-tube fertilization as a guest speaker before the annual meeting of the American Association of Anatomy in Madison, Wisconsin. It was "a great joy," one of the few she would know.

Meanwhile, Valy's academic career continued to be troubled as did the marriage. Miriam finally left him, taking the children with her to New York. As if her marital distress was not more than enough to cope with, her second child Lucy became a heartbreaking problem. Although the symptoms had not been noticeable when Lucy was a baby, by the time she was school age she was afflicted with severe muscular and neurological problems, including epilepsy. She was wracked with grand mal seizures, her speech thick and halting. Her physical handicaps gave the impression that she was mentally retarded, which was in no way true. To the contrary she was mentally agile and sensitive, which made her all the more vulnerable to rejection by schoolmates. After a while, Lucy refused to go to school anymore. Lucy was stronger than her mother; Miriam could not force her to go. The truant officer was constantly after Lucy and threatening her mother with court action. Miriam fled across the New York border into Connecticut to get Lucy away from New York school authorities. Although Miriam received three job offers from research laboratories in New York, she could accept none of them.

Their situation was becoming increasingly untenable when fate intervened again. "It was a time when things were so bad, I don't think I could have continued living if I didn't think that someday I'd go back to work with Rock on the fertilization of eggs, again." Short of that, he had given her permission to undertake the research on her own whenever and wherever she could. She applied for a fellowship at Bryn Mawr to study new techniques for staining and preserving cells. To get it she needed recommendations from people familiar with her work and abilities. Harried by her home situation, she didn't have time to write Rock for a reference. So, in a highly unusual gesture, she telephoned him. It proved to be the most fortuitous call she would ever make. "Had I written him, I would only have asked for the recommendation, but by phoning him, he asked all about what was going on in my life," Miriam noted. "Had we not talked together, I would never have told him."

He was appalled that Miriam — that any woman, for that matter — had to fend for herself and her children. Rock, recognizing perhaps more clearly than she, how desperate her situation was, urged her to rejoin his research staff as quickly as she could. Beyond having her on his staff, he also wanted to have her near enough so that he could be of personal help to her. She rejoiced in the offer.

Her yearning to again take up the test-tube-conception work was to go unfulfilled, however. When she returned to his laboratory early in 1952, she found Rock's research was taking totally new directions. From time to time he indulged Miriam's and his own interest in test-tube fertilization by providing her with ovarian tissue and permitting her to attempt it. But the work was never again a primary focus of research in Rock's laboratory. Actually, she succeeded with it once more, but didn't "bother" to report it. She came over time to feel that it was pressure from the Catholic community and, indirectly, a more subtly expressed coolness by the hospital administration that dissuaded Rock from pursuing it further.

Part of the reason Miriam returned to Rock was that she had heard there were special school arrangements in Boston for children with Lucy's problems. Rock arranged for her to work on an hourly basis, any hours she chose. She would come to the laboratory in the morning after Lucy went to school and leave at three to be home when Lucy returned. "Lucy slept ten hours a night and I slept five, so I worked those five hours when she was asleep, writing and typing at home." Lucy's school attendance was very erratic. Rock allowed Miriam to bring Lucy to the lab. She would play with crayons and paper, and later a little TV set, at one side of the room while her mother worked nearby. It was not as benign an arrangement as it appeared on the surface. Lucy could be very bothersome to people who were not used to her behavior. Due to her neurological disorder, she would have outbursts of temper and peevishness. Her epileptic seizures were a constant concern, for fear she would injure herself on the hospital premises. To Miriam, they became so commonplace they no longer upset her or interfered with her routine. The two became familiar figures walking each morning up the hill to the Free Hospital.

Rock knew all too personally himself the economic hardship that underlay many of Miriam's decisions to keep Lucy with her so much of the time. She could not afford a baby-sitter, and Lucy would become so obstreperous if her mother did not take her everywhere with her that no baby-sitter would stay with her. To stretch their income, they would eat their meals at the Free Hospital cafeteria, walk to work or school, attend free lectures and do little else. Miriam's slender tether to professional life became the time in the laboratory or library. After a while, even the small apartment became too much to manage. Moreover, landlords did not look kindly on this woman, grown misshapen and drably dressed, or her daughter who took "fits" all the time. No matter how complicated the arrangements were that she had to make to see that Lucy was properly cared for, Miriam also managed to get the work done. One summer, after she'd miraculously found a place for Lucy and her to stay with a family at a South Shore beach, Miriam discovered there was no public transportation for her to commute to Brookline. "Dr. Rock and Dr. Mulligan had an important paper to get out and there I was stuck in Nantasket. So, Dr. Mulligan brought the work and a typewriter down to me and I did the work there on the beach." Another time, when Rock was preparing a major lecture to be given in England, Miriam had gotten so far behind in her literary research for it that she moved to a hotel next door to the Boston Medical Library. "I'd had a little insurance left to me and I spent most of it on that hotel. I was paying eleven dollars a night. Lucy would sleep late and I'd go to the library and put in a few hours work. My sister thinks that I'm crazy, but it was really just my greatest pleasure."

Lucy grew to be physically enormous and Miriam, though far smaller in stature, became heavyset. She gave little thought or attention to her own well-being or appearance. She lost her teeth because she "didn't have time to bother with the dentist," and probably not the money either. Yet, traces of her early beauty remain in her delicate hands and magnificent eyes. "All I remember about Mrs. Menkin from the early days," Rock recalled, "is that she was beautiful. Oh yes, slim and lovely. Mrs. Rock said that when she first met her, she was the prettiest girl she'd ever seen. She had the handsomest face. She's never taken pride in her housekeeping. She'd tell you that herself. But she has a phenomenal brain. Her mind is such that everything is catalogued right to the minute. Between me and Lucy and that husband of hers, she's had a very hard life. She's an absolute saint."

As Rock became immersed in work on the pill, Miriam's role remained vital, though no longer central. She served as the laboratory pivot around which the plotting of the research and testing strategies turned. She was the behind-the-scenes reference researcher and manuscript editor for scientific articles that reported the stages of its development. For Rock, she also acted as editor for the many research articles he had published on his multiple phases of research. She was equally good when he was beset by lay publications to turn out popular pieces on the pill and its role in curbing runaway birth rates. During their last years together, she became his right hand. She monitored his appointment book, typed his letters, often composing parts of them from his handwritten rough notes. She reminded him of unfinished business matters and personal duties. His work, in effect, became nearly her entire world.

After 1956, when he had to retire from the active staff at the Free Hospital, he moved his laboratories out of the hospital and into a small hospital-owned building across the street at 77 Glen Road. In it, he founded the independent Rock Reproductive Clinic. There were times when he allowed Miriam and Lucy to live there, to the consternation of the hospital superintendent, Miss Lillian Grahn. Despite her protests that their overnight stays in the building violated all hospital safety codes, Rock let them stay. He bent the rules to the breaking point, but he simply could not put them out.

When she was seventy, her son Gabriel (who had elected to live with his father, but was attentive to his mother's plight) took steps to secure Social Security allotments that had long been her and Lucy's due. By that time, she was working for Rock only as a long-distance editorial researcher. With both her and Lucy's health declining, she told him she could no longer continue on a regular basis. She still stays in close contact, mostly by phone, still occasionally looking up a reference for him and more frequently sending him items of mutual interest, clipped from her readings. Financially, she survives on her and Lucy's Social Security income. It amounts to more money, she says wryly, than she was ever paid.

Only in 1979 was she willing to have his files taken from the small three-room apartment where she and Lucy live to the rare books section at the world-famed Countway Medical Library to be catalogued for posterity. All the original records are there now, including the original ledgers on their test-tube-conception work. They are among thirty cartons of papers that attest to every aspect of Rock's career. Slowly the papers are being sorted under the expert hand of curator Richard Wolfe. Eventually they will be preserved in the Countway archives, a magnificent architectural sanctuary outfitted with temperature and humidity controls to protect its priceless collections.

Across the street, Miriam and Lucy live at best a marginal existence amidst abject furnishings, chilled by drafts and faulty radiators in winter and sweltering in the summer's heat. In the living room, there is a massive desk. On it a phone, a plastic glass of stubby pencils, a Kleenex box, scissors, and a magnifying glass. Ranged around the room are old khaki-colored file cabinets, the headboard of a bed fashioned with a bookshelf, an odd bureau, and shopping bags containing bits and pieces of mementos of their lives and fragments gleaned from the research years. A tiny manila holder, always at hand's reach, holds copies of photographs of the original test-tube-fertilized eggs.

She and Lucy make a life together that has its small joys. They often reminisce about the golden years they spent with Rock. Interspersed in their conversations are loving remarks, tenderly expressed. They are quite alone.

Without question, Miriam was an all-important woman in Rock's professional life. She was always there, to be his extra eyes, ears, hands and his most devoted bench worker. But in the 1950s another woman was to enter his research life, a woman more strange and powerful than fiction could ever invent. The curtain was descending on his basic, clinical research. It was about to rise again on an entirely new drama. The stage was being reset for the debut of a new star — the world's first oral contraceptive.

6

THE "MOTHERS" OF THE PILL

THE idea of a pill to prevent pregnancy had many fathers, grand-fathers, and even great-grandfathers. One could even say it had various uncles and other contributory male progenitors. But there is no question the pill had only two women in its lineage. Two women stand by themselves as the indisputable mothers of the pill. From the moment they came on stage in the saga of its development, they took command of the scene. They did no less than *commission* the eminent male scientists who were to be the principals in its emergence, to make or find them an oral contraceptive. The women made it plain that what they wanted was a pill — like an aspirin — that would be cheap, plentiful, and easy to use. Moreover, the women virtually directed the men to be quick about it.

One of the women, the firebrand birth control advocate Margaret Sanger, through forty years of campaigning worldwide for contraception, had already created the climate for acceptance of such a pill. At a crucial moment, she provided new impetus for the work. The other woman, in the towering person of Katherine Dexter McCormick, supplied the wherewithal: a fresh supply of money and lots of it, fresh connections, and fresh commitment. Singlehandedly, she financed the entire research effort, including extensive field trials that brought the pill into being. She knew what she wanted; she found out where to get the work done and by whom. She ordered it, paid for it, and got it. Not a single penny of government money was invested in the pill. Mrs. Mc-

Cormick laid out more than two million dollars without reservation. She would have and could have put up ten times as much, if necessary.

They made a strange pair, Margaret and Katherine. Mrs. Sanger was a petite, stylish, sweet-faced woman driven by flights of nervous energy. Her appearance and manner completely belied her steely determination and utterly free sense of sexuality. Coquettish and vain in many ways, she had three husbands and openly, at least four famous lovers. Born Maggie Higgins in 1879 and early in life a renegade Catholic, she was called everything from saint to devil. According to her biographer, Madeline Gray, Sanger was "a woman who did more for other women than anyone who ever lived." She burned with two flames. One was birth control as the birthright of all women, but particularly the impoverished, brutalized tenement women caught up in the Industrial Revolution. The other was sexual freedom for women on a par with men. "I love being ravaged by romances," she wrote in a 1914 journal. One of her early disciples wrote of her: "It was she who introduced us all to the idea of Birth Control and it, along with other related ideas about sex, became her passion. She was the first person I ever knew who was openly an ardent propagandist for the joys of the flesh." Both those passions earned for Margaret Sanger a virtually unprecedented torrent of public abuse. She became a despised target of prudery, religious prejudice, and frank male chauvinism.

Mrs. McCormick was Sanger's opposite in almost every way, except on the subject of birth control about which they shared single-minded zeal. Sanger's father had been an improvident, free-thinking socialist, a self-trained gravestone carver. Katherine, however, was born in 1875 into an aristocratic family in the town of Dexter, Michigan, founded by her grandfather. Her father was Wirt Dexter, a famous Chicago attorney, and the family ancestry in America went all the way back to 1642. They had New England roots and an unbroken succession of Harvard and Harvard Law School ties. Her mother was Josephine Moore Dexter of West Springfield, Massachusetts. Her father recognized Katherine's rare intelligence and though he died before his dream was fulfilled, he encouraged her to enroll at Massachusetts Institute of Technology. She received her Bachelor of Science degree majoring in biology from MIT in 1904 — one of the first women ever to graduate from the school. Later the same year, in a lavish wedding in Geneva, she married Stanley McCormick, the youngest son of Cyrus McCormick, inventor of the reaper and founder of International Harvester Company. Stanley had graduated with honors from Princeton in 1895 and was succeeding both as an artist and young executive in his father's firm. Within two years of their marriage, however, he became a hopeless schizophrenic and was declared legally insane. His young bride withdrew from the brilliant society in which they moved and lived thereafter as a semirecluse.

As a young woman, she was a striking beauty, statuesquely nearly six feet tall. Her husband's terrible illness, however, destroyed all interest in her own appearance. Throughout the rest of her life, she dressed in the ankle-length clothing of 1904, her bridal year. It was as if wearing the sweeping skirts and oversized hats of the Teddy Roosevelt era would retain for her some vestige of the happiness she had then known. Their wedding had been held at her mother's magnificent Château de Prangins in Switzerland, originally built for Joseph Bonaparte. For years after her husband's mental illness was confirmed, they summered at the château and wintered at first in her mother's fashionable Boston townhouse at 393 Commonwealth Avenue. Soon, however, she had built an equally sumptuous castlelike estate, called Riven Rock, at Montecito in Southern California. There, she hoped, the quiet surroundings might calm her husband. She employed forty gardeners to ensure that his environment was always beautiful and six musicians to play for him, an early manifestation of the idea that music was therapeutic for psychotics. It was all to no avail. Though immensely wealthy her life with him carried hideous personal consequences. Sanger biographer Madeline Gray discloses: "They [Katherine and Stanley] had no children, and since the Mendelian theory that madness could be inherited had recently been revived, Katherine resolved that they never would have any. Still, since he was very demanding, she undoubtedly continued to have marital relations with him." This went on for nearly forty years until his death in 1947 at age seventy-three.

Her husband's mental derangement, however, led Katherine to Hudson Hoagland, the co-founder of the Worcester Foundation for Experimental Biology, and through him, to Gregory Pincus and John Rock. Katherine spent a great deal of money over the years in a search for a cure for her husband's schizophrenia. In 1927, she established the Neuroendocrine Research Foundation. Though its offices and animal research were at Harvard Medical School, its principal human studies went on at the Worcester State Hospital for indigent mental patients. There, Hudson Hoagland, whose research field was neurophysiology — the electrochemical phenomena of mental activity, normal and abnormal — was collaborating on the use of adrenal hormones to treat schizophrenia. Though the therapy never worked, Katherine developed great respect for Hoagland.

As soon as her husband died, she ended her support for psychiatric research. She had something else in mind. Her financial hands were still not completely untied, but soon would be. For decades her father-in-law had been trying to regain control of the millions he had regularly been passing along to his son. Katherine, however, fought and won for her rightful inheritance when Stanley died. By 1952 she had her money in hand. She'd sold off five estates, including Riven Rock, to pay inheritance taxes and reduce her fixed expenses. She was ready to move on the project that now consumed her: "to achieve a fool-proof contraceptive, which is the main end I hold in view at present, and over which I chafe constantly."

She laid the groundwork for what she planned to do even before she completed straightening out her finances. Late in 1950, she took the first steps. She recontacted her former acquaintance, Margaret Sanger. Katherine had given token financial support to contraceptive research funded through the Planned Parenthood Federation over the years, and had allowed Margaret Sanger to use the Geneva château for an international World Population Conference in 1927. But most of Katherine's feminist energies had gone into women's suffrage, which Margaret denigrated as a "superficial reform." Intermittently, the two women had corresponded for twenty years over the possibility of a major contraceptive breakthrough.

In October 1950, Katherine wrote to Margaret to ask her opinion on "two questions that are very much with me these days." They were: "A) Where you think the greatest need of financial support is today for the National Birth Control Movement; and B) What the present prospects are for further birth control research, and by research I mean contraceptive research." Margaret lost no time in replying, "I consider that the world and almost our civilization for the next twenty-five years is going to depend upon a simple, cheap, safe contraceptive to be used in poverty stricken slums, jungles and among the most ignorant people." Margaret proposed $25,000 a year to start, divided among five or six universities, "definitely to be applied for contraceptive control."

Mrs. McCormick had other ideas. She had little confidence in academic approaches to research. She wasn't interested in advancing fundamental knowledge. She wanted results. To Hoagland's surprise she burst into his office unannounced one day in 1950, demanding to know, "What are we going to do about it?" He assumed she still had schizophrenia in mind and began to bring her up to date on his current research into the biology of madness. No, no, no, she interrupted him. She was not talking about that problem. What she meant was the impending world population crisis! Though surprised by her sudden change of interest, Hoagland informed her he could help. He would call in his colleague, Gregory Pincus, an expert in the field of mammalian reproduction. In fact, Mrs. McCormick already had familiarized herself with Pincus's work and was just going through the amenities with Hoagland.

Meanwhile Margaret was doing her homework with Pincus, too. There is no record of the fateful meeting between Sanger and Pincus, but it was in January or February 1951. He accepted an invitation to dine at her Manhattan apartment with Margaret and her friends, gynecologists Hannah and Abraham Stone, who had fought for birth control by her side in New York since the mid-1920s. Margaret beseeched Pincus "in the name of womanhood to rally the world of science" in a now-or-never effort to come up with a solution for contraception. According to later reports, Pincus told her that the realization of such a contraceptive was not unthinkable, "but such an undertaking would require money to purchase all of the material, engage staff, and obtain thousands of rats and rabbits." He was somewhat taken aback when Mrs. Sanger said the best she could offer him to begin was a paltry $2,500. But Pincus was ambitious and he also saw in the challenge a chance to show his academic enemies at Harvard, who had treated him outrageously years earlier, what he could really do. He was absolutely confident he could turn the scientific trick Mrs. Sanger so frantically wanted. She correctly sensed that people found existing birth control approaches outmoded, disagreeable, cumbersome, and inadequate. She felt that a brand-new approach was the only way to keep the birth control movement viable.

One legend holds that while driving back to Shrewsbury alone in his car, the idea upon which a contraceptive pill could be based struck Pincus like the proverbial bolt out of the blue. Another version, far more likely, was that he went back to the Worcester Foundation and thought about it long and hard. Up to that point in his life, Pincus had no interest in contraception or world population problems. But he was a consummate scientist and in his field, many felt, he had no peer. One thing is certain: he recalled a scientific article written nearly

twenty years earlier, which had impressed him at the time. It reported
a very limited experiment, but one, nonetheless, that showed the sex
hormone progesterone could prevent female rabbits from releasing an
egg. What Pincus did not know at the time was that John Rock already was using progesterone (and estrogen) in live women and obtaining that contraceptive effect. Rock's purpose, however, was not to
prevent conception but to try to achieve it. Neither man knew of the
other's research line though they were only forty miles away from one
another.

Both men were drawing on a small, but steadily growing body of
knowledge. All scientific work builds on previous discoveries, of
course, and the pill was no exception in that regard. What made it
unique was the speed with which it emerged once the goal was set.
Before that could come about, however, the basic physiology of the
female reproductive cycle had to be understood. Even when that was
known, a new form of the cycle-governing hormones had to be devised, for natural sex hormones are ineffective if swallowed. They only
work when injected.

In the long view the genesis of the pill began in 1890 when a
Viennese gynecologist, Emil Knauer, showed that the ovaries somehow govern the development of female sex characteristics. By trans-
planting mature ovaries into immature or castrated young female animals, he found they rapidly developed mature sex characteristics.
Knauer suggested with great foresight that some sort of "generative
ferment" was going on; a ferment worked by some unknown secretion
from the ovary that was carried to the reproductive tract by the blood
stream. He was right. The secretion, of course, later proved to be
female sex hormones.

By 1921, the first suggestion appeared that an extract from the
ovaries of pregnant animals might work as a contraceptive for women,
by inhibiting ovulation. Ludwig Haberlandt, an Austrian physiologist,
found that an animal became sterile if he transplanted into its pelvis
an ovary from an already-pregnant animal. While no one yet knew
what the ovarian substance was, Haberlandt went so far as to postu-
late that someday it might be available and could be taken orally by
women. He contended it would be more effective in preventing pregnancies than anything then known.

Two scientists at the University of Rochester in New York, Drs.
George W. Corner, Jr. and Willard M. Allen, identified the intriguing
ovarian hormone in 1928. They found that it both prepared the womb

for pregnancy and sustained pregnancy. Therefore, they named it progesterone combining the Latin, *pro* (meaning in favor of) and *gestare* (to bear). Meanwhile, other investigators had discovered that the source of progesterone was the corpus luteum, the peculiar "yellow body" formed from the empty follicle following release of an egg. During pregnancy, a continuous high level of progesterone prevents any more eggs from ripening. Pregnant women do not ovulate.

The feminizing hormone (whose presence Knauer had surmised) was identified in 1929 by Edward Doisy at Washington University in St. Louis. When he treated rats with follicle liquid extracted from pig ovaries, the rats rapidly became receptive to mating. Doisy named the hormone estrogen, from the Greek *oistros* (meaning frenzy or mad desire) and *gennein* (to beget).

Most startling, however, was the discovery in 1926 by Philip E. Smith of Columbia that male and female sex glands are governed not only by their own self-produced hormones, but by others — from the brain. Smith transplanted fragments of fresh tissue from the anterior pituitary, a marble-sized organ beneath the base of the brain, into immature rats and mice. They matured sexually, quickly and very precociously. Reversing the experiment bolstered the evidence. When the pituitary gland was removed, rats of both sexes lost their sex function. The work strongly suggested, and it was later shown, that the pituitary and indeed the hypothalamus gland that arises on an adjoined axis in the midbrain have constant and intimate interplay with the primary sex glands.

The question for years was how do they "talk" to one another from such distant locations within the body? The answer came with the understanding of the "feedback mechanism." Biologically, the feedback process describes a communication loop, roughly comparable to an on-off light switch. In living systems, the on-off switches are high or low levels of hormones. In other words, a high level of one hormone signals the production of another, which in turn shuts off the production of the first — and vice versa. In women, in a simplified sense, the feedback loop for the menstrual cycle begins with a low level of both estrogen and progesterone. The low level of estrogen "tells" the pituitary gland to make FSH (follicle stimulating hormone). The stimulated follicle makes more estrogen. A rising level of estrogen then "tells" the pituitary to also make some LH (luteinizing hormone). As all three hormones — estrogen, FSH, and LH — reach a given quantity, a single egg is ripened and released. LH then converts the empty follicle into a corpus luteum, a miniature progesterone factory. The corpus luteum then pours out progesterone and the ovary continues to make estrogen. As the amounts of these two hormones peak, their quantity turns off FSH and LH production back in the pituitary.

But, what if pregnancy occurs? How will the pituitary gland in the brain know and respond? The newly created placenta, itself, produces a messenger hormone, HCG (human chorionic gonadatropin) which will "tell" the ovary a new human life is forming. HCG instructs the ovary to keep the corpus luteum functioning to produce more progesterone and also instructs the ovary to continue making estrogen. If no pregnancy occurs, no message is sent or received. Then, the corpus luteum lives for only fourteen days and scars over. With the demise of the corpus luteum, progesterone production plummets. Estrogen production also drops markedly. Briefly, the whole female sex hormone system shuts down. The womb, having received no life-supporting instructions from the hormones, sheds the soft, velvety lining it had readied to receive a conceptus. The shedding is the monthly bleeding of menstruation. The bottom-level of estrogen once again signals the pituitary to begin the cycle anew.

Had conception occurred, a different reproductive scenario would have played out. The corpus luteum pumping out progesterone would have blocked the "feedback" cycle. A continuous high level of progesterone would suppress the cycle, thus preventing any further emission of eggs by the ovary. Nature, in effect, confers a temporary sterility against additional pregnancies, so that one pregnancy is not superimposed on another. If a woman breast-feeds her newborn, a similar egg-free period also persists for several months following delivery. Again, this naturally "safe" period is provided to protect her from the burden of a new pregnancy until the suckling baby is weaned.* Where there is no egg, no conception is possible.

In 1937, a Columbia University gynecologist, Raphael Kuzrok, first observed the ovulation-free monthly cycles in breast-feeding women. He noted such cycles also occasionally occur in normal, fertile women. "If such cycles could be produced at will," he ventured, "we would have available a safe contraceptive method." The same year, three University of Pennsylvania scientists, A. W. Makepeace, G. L. Weinstein, and M. H. Friedman, proved — in animals — that this was

---

* This breast-feeding period, however, varies from woman to woman and is not considered a reliable form of birth control for long periods of time.

achievable. They showed that highly fertile mated female rabbits* indeed did not ovulate after they were given injections of progesterone. This was the science report that flashed back into Pincus's mind when he was rummaging around for a clue for a new contraceptive.

The University of Pennsylvania team's discovery of the potential of progesterone in suspending ovulation had no practical use at the time. Pure progesterone was available only from human and animal extracts and cost approximately $5,000 an ounce. Moreover, it had to be administered by injection to be effective. Yet, they had proven that progesterone was a key substance that could be used to suspend ovulation by jamming the feedback system. Manipulation of estrogen, it was found, could do the same thing. But high levels of estrogen were later to become associated with increased risk of breast, uterine, and cervical cancers.

Within the interruption of the feedback loop governing the reproductive cycle lay the physiologic basis for birth control. This became apparent in 1945 to Harvard and Mass. General Hospital endocrinologist Fuller Albright. He clearly saw how estrogen and/or progesterone could achieve egg-free menstrual cycles. He called it "birth control by hormone therapy." That year in an essay that became known retrospectively as Albright's Prophecy, he expounded a concept of birth control that was exceedingly close to the regimen ultimately employed with the pill:

> Since preventing ovulation prevents pregnancy, one could employ the same principles on birth control. Thus, for example if an individual took 1 milligram of diethylstilbesterol [synthetic estrogen] by mouth daily from the first day of her period for the next 6 weeks, she would not ovulate during the interval; if she wanted to continue the birth control further, she could continue the stilbesterol and take a course of progesterone to cause menstruation. . . . One could juggle the above therapeutics to make the menstrual period come on the least undesirable day.

(In a National Science Foundation study of the innovative process in science, the question is raised why Albright's suggestions were not quickly pursued. Later, stilbesterol was linked to certain cancers in

---

* Rabbits ovulate only on mating — to test progesterone-suppression of ovulation, therefore, the rabbits have to be mated before they are given injections.

women. Progesterone was expensive and had to be injected. But "perhaps even more important this suggestion was made in an obscure journal (*Essays on Biochemistry*) with only limited readership.")

Albright's study focused primarily on relief of serious menstrual disorders and only secondarily considered the contraceptive effect of the hormones. This was politically a far safer posture in the anti–birth control climate of Massachusetts. The 1944 referendum to ease the ban on birth control was followed by another in 1948. Both were voted down. Clearly there was a stone wall of social resistance at the time against birth control. Another point of contention was the ethical question of whether a medicine could rightly be used for a nontherapeutic purpose. This had simply never come up before and it was a vexatious idea. Thus, though the rationale for using female sex hormones to suspend fertility was known by the mid-1940s, no move was made to exploit the information for nearly another generation.

But the real roadblock was the lack of a cheap, orally effective form of progesterone. Here, too, however, advances in science were beginning to fill in some essential pieces of the puzzle. A new era of steroid chemistry was dawning. Without it, the pill could not have been born. The word steroid means "like a sterol." Sterols usually are solid alcohols (with some exceptions when they are liquid) that are abundant in plants and animals. The most familiar is cholesterol, which among its other purposes, also serves as the raw material for all sex hormones, male and female. All steroid hormones are essential to life; sex hormones because they maintain the species, or adrenal hormones because they maintain the individual by regulating the way the body sustains itself. In its purest form, a steroid is a crystalline, usually whitish powder. To understand the development of the pill it is essential to know that all steroids share a common molecular skeleton. That structure consists of four interconnected rings, composed of seventeen atoms of carbon. Other atoms of carbon plus hydrogen, and occasionally oxygen, are usually bonded to the rings, but lie outside them in side chains.

In 1928, a German chemist, Adolf Windaus, was awarded the Nobel Prize for figuring out molecular structure of a steroid (cholesterol).* One of Windaus's students, Adolf Butenandt, in 1939 shared the Nobel Prize with the Swiss chemist Leopold Ruzicka for their discovery of how to manipulate the cholesterol steroid. They found they could

---

* The structure later was proven inaccurate and Windaus corrected his finding.

change it into a synthetic duplicate of the male hormone, testosterone. Butenandt also first synthesized estrogen. A new era in drug development began with those discoveries. No longer was it a matter of looking for natural substances that could remedy a sickness. Suddenly, drugs could be designed to do what was wanted.

Next, the most extraordinary, marvelously eccentric American chemist, Russell E. Marker, was to enter the scene. He turned to botany for simpler sources of progesterone and found what he wanted in a species of wild yam in Mexico. It contained a basic precursor substance, which he called diosgenin. Marker found a way to transform diosgenin into a synthetic progesterone. Working in an abandoned potter's shed with makeshift equipment, in 1943 he converted some ten tons of the yam root into four and one-half pounds of synthetic progesterone. It was worth about $160,000 at the going market price. With two Mexican chemists, he formed Syntex Corporation, the name derived from *synt*hetic and M*exico*. What he did was chemically chop off a side chain of the diosgenin molecule and then treat it in a way to chemically simulate progesterone. Though the irascible Marker quarreled with his partners and walked off from the company, his replacement, Dr. George Rosenkranz, soon figured out the secret process. Overnight, Syntex became a major source of synthetic progesterone for American and international drug houses. The price dropped from eighty dollars a gram in 1941 when Marker first produced it to eighteen dollars a gram when Syntex first mass-produced it, to forty-eight cents a gram in 1952 when Syntex sold it by the ton.

Even with Marker's synthetic progesterone now plentiful and cheap, the drawback remained that, except at whopping doses, it had to be injected to be effective. Any change in the molecular structure of progesterone was believed to lower the hormone's potency. A single, but revolutionary, clue challenging that belief was uncovered by University of Pennsylvania chemistry professor Maximillian Ehrenstein. In April 1944, he reported that the structure of progesterone* could be changed — without sacrificing its effect. He bent a progesteronelike steroid molecule, giving it a different configuration, that strengthened its action. Exactly how he did it is fundamental to the story of the pill.

---

* As a steroid, progesterone has seventeen carbon atoms in the four basic rings, plus four others (in positions 18 through 21) in side chains. The molecule also has thirty hydrogen atoms and two oxygen atoms. Its formula then can be written $C_{21}H_{30}O_2$.

Ehrenstein knocked out the molecule's number 19 carbon atom, replacing it with a hydrogen atom. In the shorthand of the steroid chemist, he created a 19-nor progesterone — "nor" meaning less or minus.
Unfortunately, he was only able to extract a minuscule amount of the
new 19-nor progesterone, barely enough to test on two rabbits. In
one, however, the new steroid changed the lining of its womb exactly
as the natural hormone would have. When mated, the rabbit did not
become pregnant. In its altered form, the progesterone had suspended
ovulation in the rabbit. The dose was tiny, but the effect large enough
to suggest the substance was at least twice as potent as pure or synthetic progesterone. Ehrenstein's find broke totally new ground, but
his material had been excruciatingly difficult to purify. No one followed up on it.

Some progress also had been made stepping up the action of male
hormones so they could be taken orally — and also, which gave them
(female sex hormones) progestational activity. The problem was that
these altered hormones contained masculinizing effects when used to
treat female menstrual disorders.

That was pretty much the status of the physiology of human reproduction and the biochemistry of female sex hormones when Pincus
took up the gauntlet laid down by the two indomitable feminists,
Sanger and McCormick, to find them a birth control pill. Pincus had
kept pace with the advances in both fields and had added to them.
Gregory Goodwin ("Goody") Pincus was a broodingly handsome man,
with dark, deep-set piercing eyes. Born in Woodbine, New Jersey, in
1903 of Russian Jewish parents, his family, including two uncles,
were agronomists. When he began his studies at Cornell, he intended
to become a pomologist, an apple specialist. His intellectual interests
soon deepened into genetics and embryology. His protégé Chang believed Pincus's fascination with genetics was sparked, in part, by his
own inherited defect; he was color blind. But he also possessed a
photographic memory and could read a book at triple the speed of an
average reader. Eventually his scientific interests merged into a lifetime fascination with the entire spectrum of reproduction: the egg,
the nature of fertilization, sperm penetration, the timing and hormonal
conditions of the union, and the implantation of the conceptus in the
womb.

Pincus had gone on from Cornell to Harvard for his Ph.D. and
stayed on as a junior member of the faculty. There he made a name
for himself with his scientific colleagues and also with the public. Using

chemical and mechanical means he enticed rabbit eggs to grow and divide, thereby reportedly producing fatherless rabbits. His brilliant achievement was cited in 1936 by the university as part of its tercentenary celebration. Pincus's parthenogenetic rabbits, however, cost him dearly. He got caught in the middle of some in-house power politics at Harvard which, Hoagland says, "included some anti-Semitism and jealousy." At any rate, Pincus was not reappointed to the Harvard faculty. Fortunately, he was allowed to spend the last year of his faculty term at the Strangeway Laboratory in Cambridge, England.

It was also fortunate that Pincus had met Hoagland while the two men were at Harvard. Hoagland had his quarrels with Harvard, too, and had moved along to Clark University to head a small biology department there. When Pincus's England stint was ending with no further job prospects in sight, Hoagland offered Pincus a courtesy appointment on the Clark faculty, but had to raise private funds to pay his salary. The most important venture to emerge from the two men's friendship and scientific alliance was the Worcester Foundation for Experimental Biology, which they co-founded as an independent, private, nonprofit research institution in 1944. At first, it was a two-man operation. During the lean years, Hoagland cut grass and Pincus looked after the lab animals. But they created for themselves the opportunity they wanted, a place to devote full time to research without interference and on their own impeccable standards.

While in England, Pincus also met Min-Chueh Chang, a Chinese graduate student trapped in England by the war and unable to return home. In 1945 Pincus persuaded Chang to join the fledgling staff at the Worcester Foundation, which Chang says was represented as a far more substantial operation than he found it upon his arrival. Chang was a pure basic scientist and a sperm specialist. He never fully accepted the foundation's involvement with businessmen and drug houses, even though the foundation's reputation attracted customers who wanted truly independent, unbiased, accurate work done. Chang was appalled when his first assignment at the foundation was in practical animal husbandry. He was to collect eggs from cows and mate them in the test tube with sperm from prize bulls. Then, the budding embryos could be handily shipped en masse to be implanted in local cows that would serve as surrogate mothers. It was a lot cheaper than shipping herds of cows and whole bulls. After several months Chang prevailed on Pincus to let him continue his own sperm capacitation studies with rabbits. (A gifted investigator, Chang had a fine

talent for handling exquisitely delicate male reproductive specimens.)
In 1950 Chang won an award for distinguished achievement from the
American Society for the Study of Sterility for his sperm research. As
Pincus saw their relationship, he was the egg man and Chang the
sperm man. In the view of the scientific community, Chang was the
sperm biologist *par excellence,* and Pincus, the world's foremost authority on the mammalian egg. Both their lines of research were essential to putting necessary scientific underpinnings in place for the pill.

All the players and props were now on stage for the emergence of
the pill. The final preparatory move came in 1951 when Margaret
Sanger and Katherine McCormick traveled to the Worcester Foundation. There Mrs. McCormick met Pincus for the first time. In a scene
that could match anything in fiction, according to Mrs. Pincus, the
two "ladies" told her husband they wanted quick results. They were
sure, they said, that no man was in a better position to answer the key
question: Could a physiological contraceptive be found that would
be safe for mass use and be available within the next few years? Pincus
protested that science doesn't work that way. He hedged with a qualified yes, though he couldn't guarantee it. They pressed him on the
point of how certain he would be if he were assured that there would
be adequate funding to bring all relevant information, skills, staff,
and supplies to bear on the pursuit. He thought so. Then, would he
himself undertake the project at the foundation, if he were adequately
funded? Yes, he would. Over and over, Mrs. McCormick wanted to
know when he would get started and how much it would cost. Pincus,
who had given it no calculated thought, tried to put her off. Finally,
forced by her insistence, "right off the cuff, right off the top of my
head," he said $125,000. With that Mrs. McCormick took out her
checkbook and wrote him a check for $40,000. "This is the end of
the fiscal year," she told him. "I will talk to my financial man and you
will get the rest." And he did.

At first, Mrs. McCormick funneled the money through the Planned
Parenthood Federation of America's New York office, using it as a
blind through which she could preserve her secret role. But the birth
control pill project, strangely, did not arouse much enthusiasm at the
federation. Margaret Sanger found that "they have evidently not been
sold on the Pincus research." Mrs. McCormick was especially irritated
that the federation's practice was to take 15 percent of all donations
for what was considered "international" work. Thereafter, she dealt
directly with the experts: Pincus at the foundation and Rock (when

he became involved) in Brookline, supplying the money without an intermediary. That way she also avoided any legal snarls that might have resulted from the federation's control over all patents resulting from research it sponsored.

Her commitment to the research grew as fast, according to James Reed in *From Private Vice to Public Virtue,* as Pincus could rewrite his budget. The crash program for a birth control pill moved into high gear. It would triumph in less than a decade.

7

THE PILL IS BORN

THE work began, Chang's records show, on April 25, 1951. They had no way of knowing where it would lead or how long it would take. No one could have been more amazed than they, that they were on the right track from almost the very beginning. They toyed briefly with the idea of trying to adapt Chang's sperm capacitation research, perhaps, to find a way to change women's chemical receptivity to it. But that approach was abandoned almost immediately. It didn't fit Sanger and McCormick's bill and, further, the basic science wasn't clear.

Pincus already had decided that progesterone was their best shot. So, the starting point was to try to duplicate the long-ignored experiments of Makepeace, Weinstein, and Freidman at the University of Pennsylvania, who eighteen years earlier had stopped rabbits from ovulating by injecting them with progesterone. Pincus designed the study and Chang, along with another Worcester Foundation scientist, Anne Merrill, reluctantly carried it out. There was little challenge in the work for Chang. Rather, it was a tedious, time-consuming sort of assembly-line project. Day after day, he administered progesterone to rabbits, set them to mating, and then checked to see if the females became pregnant. He also sacrificed many of them to check the effect of progesterone on their ovaries to see if egg production was halted. Chang refined the dosage and timing of the injections in scores of rabbits. He discovered that pellets of progesterone could be implanted under the female rabbit's skin to inhibit ovulation on a long-term sustained-release basis, an approach now being tested in humans with modern variations of progesterone.

It was at Chang's suggestion that the work was transferred to rats, because they are more similar than rabbits to humans in that they are spontaneous ovulators. Rabbits have to copulate to trigger ovulation. Chang repeated the regimen of progesterone injections in hundreds of rats. The progesterone that was used was, of course, the standard variety of the day, the synthetic derived from Marker's marvelous yams. Although the effect was a trifle better in the rats, when administered by mouth, the roadblock remained that to supress ovulation required huge doses. Nonetheless, the rerun of the Pennsylvania experiments reconfirmed that progesterone could work as a contraceptive — in animals.

As it soon turned out, there really was no need to do such extensive animal studies — at least not to answer that question — though Pincus did not know it at the time. Forty miles away in Brookline, John Rock was carrying on infertility studies with women patients in which progesterone was clearly preventing ovulation. Pincus and Rock had lost touch with one another during the 1940s. By chance they met at a scientific conference in 1952 and each learned what the other was up to. The timing could not have been more fortuitous.

It was at this very juncture that Rock was beginning to use synthetic progesterone to try to overcome sterility in women whose infertility defied diagnosis. Either they didn't ovulate consistently or when they did become pregnant, they immediately miscarried. Some also may have had undiagnosable forms of endometriosis. Rock theorized that for some of them their problem might be an immaturity, an underdevelopment of their Fallopian tubes or womb. If that were the case, he thought that treatment with the "hormones of pregnancy," estrogen and progesterone, might induce the desired maturing of those organs. That was what happened, he felt, during a natural pregnancy, and he thought it might work during what he blithely termed a "pseudopregnancy." He tried it on "eighty frustrated but valiantly adventuresome patients to whom the experimental nature of the treatment and its unknown but probably harmless and only possibly helpful effects were carefully explained. Like us, they wanted to try it." He put them on an unrelieved regimen of the hormones. They received doses of progesterone that were gradually increased from a low of 50 milligrams to extremely high doses of 300 milligrams. They also received estrogen daily — without letup — for three to five months in doses of 5 to 30 milligrams. Because the hormones were taken *every* day, the women did not menstruate.

Rock well knew the contraceptive effect of the treatment: "They were assured conception could not occur during the treatment. It couldn't because the hormones stopped ovulation."

One aspect of the pseudo-pregnancy upset many of the women and their husbands. It was too much like the real thing. All the classic signs of pregnancy occurred. The women did not menstruate, their breasts became tender and enlarged, and some had nausea remarkably similar to morning sickness. Since they were eager to be pregnant, it was difficult to convince them they weren't.

To Rock's delight, within four months after the treatment was concluded, an astonishingly high number of the women — thirteen — did conceive. This "felicitous" result, as Rock called it, was dubbed the "Rock rebound" effect, because the women seemingly rebounded from the pseudo-pregnancy to the real thing. Rock, however, was never certain whether the pseudo-pregnancy actually worked by maturing their reproductive systems or because the system was placed in a complete state of rest.

Although the primary purpose of Rock's study was to overcome sterility, the counterpoint was dramatically confirmed. The estrogen-progesterone regimen blocked ovulation. And Rock knew it. He knew the potential contraceptive use that was latent in the treatment as early as 1951.

To say the least, Pincus was intrigued by Rock's experiment. Pincus's interest, of course, centered on the ovulation-inhibition effect. Rock, in turn, was equally fascinated by Pincus's animal trials with progesterone alone. As a result of their chat, and at Pincus's urging, Rock decided to try progesterone alone on a new series of infertile women, much as Pincus was doing with the lab animals. Progesterone was known to be safer than estrogen and might do the job on its own. At some point, Pincus also ventured the suggestion that the progesterone be given for only twenty-one days in the menstrual cycle as was the practice in the treatment of menstrual abnormalities in the 1940s. By stopping it for a week, the menstrual flow would come in. Psychologically, that would solve the problem of raising false hopes in the barren couples taking part in the test. While the idea of cycling the progesterone in this situation was a clever one that truly served an important psychological purpose, Pincus may have had a second reason for suggesting it. When he sought supplies of synthetic progesterone from the G. D. Searle Company of Skokie, Illinois, for Rock's second trial with pseudopregnancies, Pincus was warned by Searle's chief chemist, Dr. Frank Saunders, that the company's director of biological research, Victor Drill, wanted no part of any compound that interfered with the menstrual cycle. In that era, and largely still today, doctors shy away from any tampering with menstruation, contending that it is tantamount to "going against Nature." It is a peculiar intellectual block in view of the fact that menstruation, which can be debilitating, is biologically necessary only while women are interested in childbearing.

By 1953 Rock had the progesterone-only pseudo-pregnancy experiment well under way. As in his first experiment, only women proven to be barren for at least two years were chosen. This time, each sterile volunteer had to demonstrate she ovulated regularly. Rock's old stand-by, the rhythm-temperature charting method, was used. And, once again, the "Rock rebound" phenomenon occurred. Four of the thirty women in this trial became pregnant at the end of the course of treatment. In Rock's eyes, the progesterone-only regimen was wonderfully successful insofar as finding a new aid for the relief of infertility was concerned. But the results were not as satisfying for Pincus. Rock's thoroughness in checking by indirect measures* revealed that as many as 15 percent of the women in the study showed some signs they had ovulated. Further, Rock found the chance of ovulation persisted regardless of how large the dose of progesterone was. While Rock was confident that it was appropriate to give women who were desperate to become pregnant massive doses of progesterone for a few months, it was unthinkable to consider doing it for prolonged periods as a contraceptive. Moreover, the hormone still had to be injected. It just wouldn't suffice as a contraceptive, Pincus had to concede.

The search for the cheap and easy surefire contraceptive that Sanger and McCormick had placed on order seemed stalemated. Pincus, however, was not a man to be easily dissuaded. For him, the stakes had become too high. He wanted to succeed and intended to. Earlier, he'd come close to scoring a major breakthrough in developing a tailor-made corticosteroid, only to have his work overshot by others. The natural cortisone molecule contained a baffling complexity. It

---

* The indirect measures included signs of temperature shifts at midcycle, cervical smears that reflected ovulatory changes in the vaginal secretions, and hormonal breakdown products in urine samples that are telltale signs that ovulation is occurring.

carried an inner ring of oxygen that was nearly impossible to duplicate. As a consultant to Searle, Pincus had come up with a technically
ingenious method. By flowing a corticosteroid raw material through
the adrenal gland of a sow, he could inveigle the gland to insert the
elusive oxygen atom precisely as Nature did. Just as Searle geared up
at great cost to use Pincus's method, an Upjohn Company scientist
found an elegantly simple way to do it. An innocuous bacterium could
be set to putting the oxygen atom in place in a process called micro-
biological fermentation. Pincus's approach was scuttled.

But Pincus had become very knowledgeable about steroid chemistry
and had worked as a special consultant on a contractual basis for
many pharmaceutical firms in the United States and for Syntex in
Mexico. His extensive contacts with drug houses were about to pay
off. When Rock's infertility studies with synthetic progesterone failed
to serve Pincus's search for the pill, he wrote to his contacts at all the
drug companies then doing hormone work. He asked if any of them
had anything under development that might be a stronger progesterone,
in the hope that smaller doses could be used and might work more
effectively. A glorious surprise awaited him. Two men had ready-
made what he was looking for. One was Dr. Carl Djerassi, then an
executive vice-president of the Syntex Corporation and one of its
geniuses in steroid manipulation, and the other a Searle steroid chemist,
Frank Colton. Neither man had an inkling of the contraceptive use
that their brainchildren could serve. The pill destined to change the
world as the first oral contraceptive for womankind was quite literally
invented.

Dr. Carl Djerassi is a Viennese-born chemist of outstanding reputation, now professor of chemistry at Stanford University and president
of Zoecon Corporation. He had written his Ph.D. thesis at the University of Wisconsin on a "very difficult problem in the steroid field —
namely the chemical conversion of the male sex hormone testosterone
into the estrogenic hormone, estradiol." Only twenty-six years old in
1949, he was yearning to try his hand at synthesizing new cortisones,
then the hottest subject in the steroid field. Joining Syntex in Mexico,
Djerassi performed like a virtuoso, quickly synthesizing cortisone —
the breakthrough drug houses the world over sought — via two different pathways.

In 1950, Djerassi set out to try to construct an orally effective
progesterone. To do it, he followed Ehrenstein's lead that potency
could be enhanced by altering the molecule, rather than duplicating

it. Djerassi also used a process devised in 1949 by an Australian chemist, Arthur J. Birch, at Oxford University, which simplified the elimination of the 19-nor carbon atom. He applied the Birch procedure to a misfit hybrid sex hormone he'd concocted, and the result was crystalline pure 19-nor progesterone — four to eight times as powerful as the natural form. Now, he knew he was on a hot streak. Again, there was a lead from passed-over scientific literature, he reports in his book, *The Politics of Contraception*. In 1937, a Swiss chemist, Hans H. Inhoffen, had enhanced the oral action of a synthetic form of the male hormone testosterone by tripling a carbon bond at position 17 of the molecule. The maneuver also gave the substance, called ethisterone, some mild progestational activity. It was, as Djerassi held, "the hint that we needed in the summer of 1951." Already aware that removing the 19-nor carbon atom from his own hybrid stepped up its progestational character, Djerassi found "it did not take us long" to realize that doing the same thing to Inhoffen's enthisterone (which had become commercially available in the 1940s as a treatment for menstrual difficulties, but had undesirable masculinizing side-effects over long-term use) "would increase its progestational strength . . . and not interfere with its oral effectiveness." It worked. In his book, Djerassi states: "Luis Miramontes, a young Mexican chemistry student carrying out his bachelor thesis in the Syntex laboratories under the direction of George Rosenkranz and myself, succeeded on October 15, 1951 in synthesizing 19-nor-17 alpha-ethynyltestosterone, generically known as *norestheisterone* or *norethindrone*." They had mastered it. They had built the world's first acceptable orally active high-powered synthetic progesterone. Djerassi himself said that "not in our wildest dreams did we imagine that eventually this substance" would become the active ingredient of oral contraceptives.*

To distinguish the new orally active progestational agents from Nature's own progesterone, the new substances were called *progestins* — an umbrella term for progestational substances in general. Djerassi sent a few samples out to be tested to see how they would act in living systems. The first to receive it was Dr. Roy Hertz, who coincidentally had assisted Ehrenstein on his original work with the first crude 19-nor progesterone at the University of Pennsylvania. In 1952, however,

---

* Djerassi applied for a patent on November 22, 1951, and reported the synthesis of the new 19-norethindrone at the April 1952 meeting of the American Chemical Society's Division of Medicine Chemistry in Milwaukee, Wisconsin.

Hertz was working at the National Institutes of Health at Bethesda, Maryland, just outside Washington, D.C. He found Djerassi's norethindrone to be eight times more powerful than progesterone when administered by mouth to rabbits, guinea pigs, monkeys, and, thereafter, to three women — the first on whom it was tried. As patients of Hertz at NIH Clinical Center, they received the drug for the sole purpose of trying to control grave menstrual irregularities — hemorrhagic monthly bleeding. The idea of its use as a birth control pill was not even envisioned.

Midway across the country, another drug company, G. D. Searle, had entered the progestin race. There, the firm's chief research chemist, Frank B. Colton, an alumnus of the University of Chicago and the Mayo Clinic Research Foundation, was also "looking down the same track." Djerassi has long inferred that Colton and Searle simply took advantage of Syntex's norethindrone and modified it. Colton denies it. He'd been brought to Searle to seek a novel approach to concocting a corticoid that would have fewer of the undesirable side-effects (such as salt retention) of cortisone. He, too, studied Ehrenstein's and Birch's work, which were of renewed, highly "visible" interest to chemists in the corticoid field. Colton realized the two companies, Searle and Syntex, were running neck and neck. He quickly made a number of 19-nor steroids, all primarily progestational in effect. In interviews, Colton says that the Searle chemists went on to develop "some 200 different molecules," hoping to make a super progestin, "one better than Mother Nature's." What happened, Colton says,* was that a chemist, Professor A. L. Wilds of the University of Wisconsin, and one of his students, N. A. Nelson, devised a better method for knocking out the key 19-nor carbon atom. Though they did not report the improved process until 1953, Wilds told Djerassi of it in 1950. Wilds had been Djerassi's thesis supervisor at the University of Wisconsin. Wilds also, however, told another of his students, Dr. Jack Ralls, who was one of Colton's associates. "So we were following the same research line as Djerassi at the same time," Colton said. The Searle progestin, destined to become the first pill licensed as an oral contraceptive, had a slightly different molecular structure than Djerassi's. (While also a 19-nor compound, Colton's version had a double carbon bond between positions of carbon

---

* The National Science Foundation analysis corroborates Colton's account of the development at Syntex of progestin, though Djerassi does not mention it in his book. Djerassi, indisputably, was the first to succeed.

5 and 10 on the molecule, while Djerassi's was at position 4 and 5.)
Searle called its version *norethynodrel,* and catalogued it as SC-4642,
code for Searle Company, compound number 4642. Colton filed for
Searle's patent on SC-4642 on August 31, 1953. Once again, it was
expected the compound would be used as a treatment for menstrual
disorders. Neither Searle nor Syntex had any notion that the exciting
new progestins would be fated for birth control usage.

Thus it was that when the prospects looked darkest, Pincus's queries
turned up not one but dozens of model compounds of the new progestins. They were literally sitting on the pharmaceutical companies'
shelves waiting for him. A few drug houses besides Searle and Syntex
also had new progestational compounds, but none were like Djerassi's
and Colton's. Over the course of a year or so, Searle sent Pincus some
two hundred variations. Min-Chueh Chang and Anne Merrill had their
work cut out for them anew. The rabbit and rat experiments had to be
repeated all over again, this time using the new agents. In short order,
Pincus and Chang narrowed down the many offerings to three: Syntex's
norethisterone (Djerassi's model, tagged S-759) and two from Searle,
norethynodrel (Colton's SC-4642) and another Searle progestin,
norethandrolone. The third, however, had male hormone (androgenic)
effects and was fairly quickly abandoned as a birth control agent. After
Pincus and Chang took the two most favorable contenders through
their battery of tests on rabbits and rats, and found them safe and con-
traceptively effective, it was time to see if the progestins would work
similarly on women.

Rock began the first supercautious tests with the compounds on
women in 1954. Again, they would be administered to try to help barren women conceive by "resting" the reproductive system and then,
hopefully, achieving a rebound effect. This time, however, an intensive
parallel study would go on. The women would be watched, charted,
and tested in every way possible to verify whether the trial compounds
truly stopped ovulation. Eventually fifty women were enlisted for what
historically became the first human trials with an oral contraceptive.
Most still were drawn from the Free Hospital clinics, but near the
study's end, early in 1955, some also were entered from a new base,
the newly formed Rock Reproductive Study Center, across the street
from the hospital. Rock had reached mandatory retirement age, sixty-
five, that year and had to move his practice into new quarters.

So far there had been no snags, but the stakes were far higher now.
Rock's major problem was overcrowding and overwork. His private

office and the fertility clinic had been housed in incredibly cramped quarters. He needed more room. The hospital made available to him a small two-and-one-half-storied yellow brick building that connected the stark nurses' quarters to the power plant. It was a customary practice for the Free Hospital to "carry" retiring staff members in some such fashion. In Rock's case, it was essential for the hospital to keep him on as a "consultant" because he generated a large share of the hospital's patients. While he cared for them medically himself, he referred them to colleagues for surgery. The building, for which he paid a small rent, was so dilapidated and disheveled that it was barely usable. He had no option, however, but to try to make do with it. Despite its condition, it doubled his work area.

Mrs. McCormick soon solved that problem in typical grand style. He recalled the first time she and Margaret Sanger came to see him. With stereotyped thinking, he mistook one for the other, presuming that the attractive, stylish woman would be the wealthy socialite, Mrs. McCormick, and the other, heavyset formidable-appearing matron would be the battling reformer. To his embarrassment, he discovered the reverse was true. Mrs. McCormick was very taken with Rock, impressed by his personal charm, his humility and his unyielding professionalism. She was, however, utterly appalled by the building in which his center was housed and referred to it with open disdain as "the Hovel." She gave him nearly $100,000 for renovations in 1955, a sum that was on the order of ten times more money than he had ever received even for research. Later Mrs. McCormick wrote Margaret: "He thinks the Hovel as I call it — it is that wretched little brick building — is costing too much for him to make over." She considered his time was worth far more than the added costs and insisted he go forward without delay. When she finally saw it completed in 1957, she wrote: "I went to see Dr. Rock yesterday and he and Dr. Garcia showed me all over the Hovel. I thought Dr. Rock was looking well and has done wonders with that miserable little building. He and Dr. Garcia really ought to have an installation on the scale of the Chateau de Versailles if the importance of their work were to be considered."

Rock also needed more help. He'd always had a coterie of young graduate doctors on hand as research fellows. Among those working with him during the 1953 progesterone-only studies and the first trials in 1954 with progestins was Dr. Luigi Mastroianni, a Yale graduate and a young obstetrician with an intense interest in infertility. Mastroianni moved right in at Rock's side, endearing himself to Rock professionally and personally. Looking back, Mastroianni admitted, "I don't really think I sensed the true significance of what was being done. But I remember the patients vividly and all the people involved in the progestin work. The concept of informed consent that is so talked about now, and is a legal requirement of any research project involving human volunteers, didn't exist then. But Rock practiced it [informed consent] before it was ever defined. There were always long and large discussions of the risk factors. It didn't matter that Rock had no formal guidelines, he set his own and they were high standards, indeed."

In-house, the project was dubbed the PPP — the Pincus Progesterone Project. For Mastroianni and others in Rock's laboratory at the time, it soon became more irreverently known as the "pee, pee, pee" project, because as one of his tasks, Mastrioanni had to check the twenty-four-hour urine samples of the subjects. If the women did not ovulate, one indication would be the absence in their urine of pregnandiol, a by-product of natural progesterone that is excreted. Another fellow of Rock's that year was Dr. Angelika Tsacona of Greece. Her contribution to the study, among others, was to follow up on seven patients (in addition to the group of fifty), who agreed to take the new progestin for two months prior to undergoing a scheduled hysterectomy. Her examination of tissue removed from their ovaries and womb provided incontrovertible proof that they had not ovulated while on the progestins.*

Rock's first human trials with the progestins was not quite completed early in 1955, and, of course, not yet reported anywhere. But the results were coming in right on the mark. While some 15 percent of the women in the previous trial (with standard progesterone) had ovulated, none did while taking the progestins! Rock was "gratified" that the progestins, as had both earlier synthetic progesterone studies, led to pregnancies through the rebound effect, in about the same ratio of women, 15 percent. Pincus, however, was ecstatic over the ovulation-inhibition effect. He was absolutely sure that they now had within their grasp the kind of pill the two women commissioned. Before the progestin trials at Rock's clinic were finished, Pincus and Rock set another two small clinical trials in motion, and they were discussing strategy for the next big step, field trials. (Clinical trials are a first step in which

---

* It rankled Miriam Menkin that Tsacona was given no credit in the final report of the first study of the progestins, though Mastroianni and another research fellow, Dr. John V. Kelley, are included in a footnote.

a relatively small number of test subjects are given a new drug and matched with controls, who are not. Those receiving the drug or placebo are selected on a random basis and both groups are closely and intensely monitored medically. Field trials encompass large numbers of volunteers who receive the drug being tested and are medically monitored for specific aspects of the material under study — safety, side effects and efficacy.) Rock felt more clinical trials were needed first. No conclusions could be drawn from a single study of fifty women, he knew. While he felt the progestins now ethically warranted further human trials to test their prowess directly as contraceptives (separate from infertility research), he also knew that legally he could not undertake such tests at the Free Hospital or his private clinic without risking criminal prosecution in Massachusetts. Violation of the state birth control law was a felony that carried penalties of up to five years in prison and fines of $1,000 for each instance in which contraceptive advice or aids were supplied.

Two other small and tenuous studies were undertaken, both of them set up by Pincus. One was at the University of Puerto Rico, where both Pincus and Rock had connections with the medical school dean, Dr. E. Harold Rinman. Through Rinman, they enlisted Dr. Celso-Ramon Garcia, a Manhattan-born Spanish-American and graduate of the State University of New York, who had gone to Puerto Rico to set up a department of obstetrics and gynecology at the medical school there. Today he is the William Shippen, Jr., Professor and Director of the Division of Human Reproduction in the obstetrics-gynecology department at the University of Pennsylvania Medical School. Garcia agreed to undertake the progestin study for Pincus. Rock served as medical adviser, personally examining tissue samples obtained from the volunteers and forwarded to him in Brookline. Garcia recruited twenty women medical students in Puerto Rico for the study. Some were married, some were not. They were not infertile, as Rock's subjects had been. Again, the study was somewhat disguised. It was designated a study of the progestins effect on the menstrual cycle. While that information was needed, the volunteers also were, of course, demonstrating the compounds' direct contraceptive effect.

It was one thing to lecture medical students on the subject of human sexuality and contraception within the confines of Harvard Medical School or to teach rhythm, an "approved" method, to indigent Catholic women, although both actions technically violated state law. It was quite another matter to publicly undertake large-scale clinical trials, involving hundreds of women, for the express purpose of contraception. That would flagrantly violate the law. (Pincus was not a medical doctor and could not treat — or test drugs on — patients and so the legal question did not confront him or the Worcester Foundation, the way it did Rock. Rock also was soon to be totally "on his own," outside Harvard's sphere of influence, in the Rock Reproductive Clinic.)

The questions the study asked all centered on the pills' (both progestins were used) potential for suppressing ovulation without disturbing other ovarian functions. Another purpose, insisted on by Rock, was to see if use of the pill produced any changes in the tissue of the cervix or womb that might suggest a cancerous effect — as may happen when estrogen is given "unopposed" by progesterone. When the contraceptive implications of the study became more openly known, the project lost favor with the hierarchy of the University of Puerto Rico, "largely Catholic-dominated positions," as Garcia pointed out. The real shortcomings in the study, however, were that the test group was far too small to be conclusive and the women too medically sophisticated. Their experience with the progestins could not reflect how well large and educationally limited populations of women would be able to handle it — the very women most in need of birth control. Soon, the university officials withdrew support of any further expansion of the study into field trials. In correspondence, Mrs. McCormick repeatedly refers to the study as a "flop" because of its limitations.

His participation in the project was a turning-point for Garcia, however. He joined John Rock's staff at the Rock Reproductive Center in 1955. But from the moment he came aboard the initial Puerto Rico trial, he became a vital fourth member of the quartet with Rock, Pincus, and Chang, who together would go on to prove the pill's worth as an oral contraceptive.

A second study was wholly ill-conceived. There is no question that it would violate the standards for human experimentation, according to today's guidelines. It involved twenty-three mental patients at the Worcester State Hospital, a mental institution operated by the Commonwealth of Massachusetts and located near the Worcester Foundation. The foundation had long-standing ties to the mental hospital through Mrs. McCormick, who had established the Neuroendocrine Research Foundation there in 1927. Times were hard and funds for state mental hospitals scarce, so the hospital administrator had no objections, especially when Mrs. McCormick paid to have the "experimental wards" in which the "volunteers stayed, refurbished and outfitted with comfortable furniture and cheerful accoutrement." In the mid-1950s, when Pincus wanted to test the pill on "a few patients," the hospital's director, Dr. Alexander Freeman, agreed.

Seven women and eight men were given progestin tablets for from three to five and one half months. They were all psychotics. A specious rationale, if there really was any at all, was that some women mental patients occasionally got pregnant, "by accident," though of course they were supposed to be protected from sexual intercourse at all times. To determine whether the women ovulated, their menstrual cycles were monitored and some biopsies were taken of endometrial tissue. Such biopsies in which a few snips of tissue are cut off the womb lining and extracted are at best extremely unpleasant and are usually very painful procedures. In the men's group, as would be expected when men are given female hormones, the progestin pills had a predictable sterilizing effect. But the men's mental disturbances made it difficult to impossible to even collect semen samples to measure the effects accurately. While the feminizing influence of the pill was only transitory, there are no grounds upon which such a study can be justified.

Pincus, however, was more intent than ever on establishing proof that the progestins were the birth control substances he sought. One of his reasons was the fifth conference of the International Planned Parenthood League to be held in Tokyo in October of 1955. Margaret Sanger and Katherine McCormick were tingling with frustration. They wanted to get the word out, at least to the scientific community, that a birth control pill was on the horizon, one that looked tantalizingly good. Pincus wanted the same thing. He wanted to stake his claim publicly, quickly. He had been burned in the earlier cortisone episode and did not want that to happen again. The women wanted Pincus to "float" the news of the pill at the Tokyo meeting. Pincus readily agreed to go and wanted Rock to go, too. Rock, however, would have no part of it. He felt any contraceptive claims for the progestins were wholly premature. His own 1954 "infertility" studies with the progestins had involved far too few women, he maintained, to make any elaborate claims about the pill's contraceptive worth. Ethically, he also knew, it was out of the question to present at such a meeting details of work not yet published. Most of all, he was not yet ready to call attention to the pill's contraceptive, as well as its infertility, benefits. He had good reason.

Far more than just unpopular, the idea of a birth control pill was still widely regarded as socially immoral and medically questionable. A birth control pill would be the first medicine in history given to well people solely for a social purpose. Behind closed doors at the leading medical centers of the country, including Harvard, the notion of a pill for women — just to prevent pregnancy — was not considered justified, proper, or even decent. In 1955, Rock was only a year away from mandatory retirement. At that point, he most certainly did not want to risk ostracism or jeopardize a long and distinguished career. Besides, as a prominent and respectful Catholic, he did not want needlessly to harden the opposition of his Church to a new form of birth control, if the pill was not the near-perfect agent it appeared to be. Pincus was not burdened by any of those concerns and so he and Chang attended the Tokyo meeting with their wives.

At the Tokyo meeting, the world heard the first glimmerings of the new pill. Before 150 delegates and participants — all of whom gave or heard another round of reports reflecting little hope of any new practical form of contraception — Pincus unveiled the studies. He gave details of the progestins' incredible contraceptive effect on the lab animals and made reference to similar preliminary effectiveness on women. "He [Pincus], in fact, was reporting the work done on humans by John Rock and by myself," Garcia notes, though neither of their names was mentioned. Rock was greatly irritated that his human studies were prematurely mentioned, even though Pincus couched his references to ovulation inhibition as a secondary finding. He pointed out that both Searle and Syntex progestins had been used in both the animal and human trials.

Instead of the explosive reaction that would have been expected, his presentation was received with yawns and skepticism. The only aspect that was regarded as new was the claim that these progestins worked — with great effectiveness — when taken by mouth. That was the transcendant point, but it passed by the audience as though it were insignificant, but some notice of his report was picked up by the popular press. At the Tokyo meeting, Pincus went all the way out on the scientific limb: "Much more investigation is, of course, needed, but they [the progestins] thus far are the most promising agents. We cannot on the basis of our observations thus far designate the ideal anti-fertility agent, nor the ideal mode of administration. But a foundation has been laid for the useful exploration of the problem on an objective basis. The delicately balanced sequential processes involved in normal mammalian production are clearly attackable. Our objective is to disrupt them in such a way that no physiological cost to the organism is in-

volved." In plain terms he made it clear that he was confident a progestin was at hand that would work as a birth control pill. "That objective," he declared, "will *undoubtedly* be attained by careful scientific
investigation" (italics added).

The next time that the first — and only significant — progestin
study (Rock's "infertility" women) was reported, at the thirteenth
Laurentian Conference early in 1956, the reaction was far different.
The Laurentian Conference was an annual meeting, originally organized by Pincus, which drew scientists from all over North America who
were involved in hormone research. It was a freewheeling, wide-open
critical forum for investigators pursuing new lines of research. Typical
of the era, the conference was partly sponsored and largely paid for by
major U.S. pharmaceutical companies who often got leads on new lines
of drug development from the sessions. At the 1956 meeting, the tigers
of the industry were all on hand. The word was out that Pincus and
Rock were on to something big. Still determined to downplay any premature claims, the paper, authored by Rock, Garcia, and Pincus — but
presented by Rock — was entitled "Synthetic Progestins in the Normal
Human Menstrual Cycle." It included, however, a subsection on "effects
on ovulation" on 125 treated cycles of fifty infertile women and fifty un-
treated cycles (controls) from Rock's clinic. As the clinical authority
on the work, it was Rock's reputation that was on the line. He showed
slide after slide illustrating the appearance of vaginal tissue, the condition of the womb-lining tissue, of ovarian tissue, and of urine analysis
studies. In the very deliberately worded language of his report, he only
would go as far as saying, "We are led to suspect that ovulation has
been inhibited in at least a very high proportion of cases." He made no
direct statement about the pill's obvious, overriding potential as a contraceptive. Once again, he stressed the fact that seven of the women
became pregnant following treatment. He appeared to be giving as-
surances that the pill did not harm the egg or the ovary.

With typical adroitness he parried questions from the confreres that
got close to the contraceptive potential in the work. "Oh dear, but I
had them all," he commented wryly. In his view it was vital that there
be nothing on the record that would prematurely flag the attention of
the politicians in Massachusetts who would make an anti–birth control
cause célèbre of the research. Nor did he "want to go so boldly and
flagrantly in the face of the Church. I think I was protecting Catholicism as such, rather than myself. I had a loyalty to the Church, a loy-

alty which kind of transcends belief. The time was not yet right to flaunt the contraceptive effect."

While Rock at the time of the Laurentian Conference feigned only a passing interest in what he truly knew was an out-and-out contraceptive effect of the pill, he nonetheless wanted the participants of the meeting to be aware of it. In a concluding session of the conference, a specialist from the University of Georgia finally voiced what was in everyone's mind — that in the Rock, Garcia, Pincus report, "it seems to me we have anti-ovulation!" Rock grinned when he remembered it. "I didn't say it, but I allowed them to know." The new birth control cat was all the way out of the bag, at last.

The research community and the drug industry went home from the conference knowing precisely what was afoot. Mrs. Sanger wrote to Mrs. McCormick: "At last the reports . . . are now out . . . and the conspiracy of silence is broken." The wisdom of Rock's position, however, can be seen in Mrs. McCormick's reply to Mrs. Sanger a month later; a letter that also illustrates their own suppressed bigotry: "I have seen an article (sent me by Rock) from a weekly called 'Scope' of which I had never heard. It may be an R.C. [a commonly used but demeaning abbreviation for Roman Catholic] church publication, but — in any case — the seven *naturally* infertile women who *surprisingly* become fertile five months after taking our sterility indication have been a very nice alibi for Dr. Rock, and have become a source of great amusement to all of us thereby!"

Briefly, Rock seemed to waver. Suddenly, he introduced into the quest for a "simple, easy and cheap" contraceptive a whole new line of research. He discovered an aberrant chemical in the vaginal mucus of some of his infertile patients, a chemical he thought acted against their husband's sperm. For a while he entertained the idea that this substance, if it could be isolated and identified, might prove to be a universal spermicidal agent. While he never succeeded in elucidating the substance, the work on the face of it seems an odd departure from the mainline pill research. If he had identified the mysterious chemical, its use would clearly be forbidden by the Catholic Church as the killing of the "germ of life" male component. Rock never intellectually accepted that line of Church thinking. He always considered unfertilized eggs and sperm — the overwhelming majority of which are emitted in life only to die — as merely cast-off cells, discards of Nature.

Yet there is a sense that he resisted, momentarily, proceeding with the pill work. The diversion with the vaginal chemical bought him time to think through one last time the sweeping social, moral, ethical, religious, and medical ramifications of a birth control pill. He was never overly fond of mavericks and he had no taste for martyrdom. But more important, before embarking on large-scale field trials from which there would be no turning back, Rock had to contend with his own conscience. It was his responsibility, above all others, to be certain that the pill would be harm*less,* as he expressed it. By harmless, he meant, when prescribed by a physician and its use monitored by a physician. On a deeper level, the morality of its use had to be crystal clear in his mind.

While he saw the overwhelming need to separate sex, in marriage, from the constant threat of pregnancy — to set sex free from its age-old link to procreation — he was far more aware than Pincus or any of the others involved in the project of the moralists' objections they would face regarding the alleged illicit use to which such a simple and private practice of birth control could be put.

Sex, indeed, would be set free, not only for the married, but for any woman, anywhere, anytime, with anyone. Not only would the risk of pregnancy be eliminated but, astonishingly, only the woman concerned would know. The whole control of her sexuality as well as her fertility would be placed in her hands. There would be no telltale act of preparedness associated with sex relations. Even more momentous, there would be no consequence, as before, no aftermath of an unwanted pregnancy or an abortion. It amounted to handing over to women, for the first time in history, not only total governance over their sexual behavior, but total privacy — some would say secrecy. Women's sexual prerogatives would equal men's.

Rock had always considered himself a scrupulous Catholic. The evolution of his own thinking about birth control was that initially of a conservative trying to preserve stable, sound family life. In the early years, the 1930s, the paramount reason he stood publicly for birth control was to combat the prevailing high maternal death rate. He wanted doctors to have the legal right to prescribe contraceptives for medically indicated reasons, whenever a mother's life would be placed at risk by pregnancy. In the late 1930s, he had even co-authored a handbook, *Voluntary Parenthood,* which advised against postponing pregnancy in early marriage. Already steeped in infertility problems, back then he felt it important to prove fertility right away because the older infertile couples became, the more intractable the problem, if there was any question of infertility. But his views changed with time and the onrush of runaway world population. And the evolution of his view on contraception was consistent with enlightened Catholic thinking.

He was deeply influenced by the famous French Jesuit anthropologist Pierre Teilhard de Chardin. Rock saw Teilhard de Chardin as "perhaps the greatest philosopher of our time . . . the Socrates, the Aquinas of our epoch, and, like them in their day, denied by blind men in high places." Teilhard de Chardin's writings not only accepted Darwin's concepts of evolution but also tried to converge science and religion. The books had been suppressed by the Vatican throughout the author's life. Rock particularly subscribed to Teilhard de Chardin's fundamental thesis, that Mankind, in its continued socialization, was struggling, evolving to a higher plane "onward and upward toward its goal: Truth." In that context, unbridled reproduction came to represent in Rock's mind "a whirlpool of destruction." Rock noted, "Man, as Father Teilhard de Chardin reminds us, is not a beast. As an animal, he too copulates, but not being a beast, and endowed with intellect, man rejects his humanism if he procreates by ignorance, by carelessness or without good intention." Rock concluded that it was consistent with Teilhard de Chardin's thinking that "parents . . . must use one or another of the available methods to render nonprocreative those numerous marital acts which properly [are] the healthful exercise of sexual function."

It was not until the late 1940s, when Rock began to perceive (along with many social scientists and demographers) the threat to social order posed by overpopulation, that he became an ardent advocate of small families.

In Rock's own lifetime, however, the death rate had plummeted. The average life expectancy was only slightly more than forty years in 1880 in America and other countries with a reasonable standard of living. Today the average lifespan is nearly eighty years, almost double what it was when Rock was born. While a boon to mankind, the incredible prolongation of life, a phenomenon wrought by improved sanitation, immunization, insect control, and antibiotics, contributed directly to the population dilemma.

While the death rate was dropping, worldwide the growth rate was steadily climbing. A sudden and intense quickening of the rate of population growth occurred in the post–World War II era. From 1945 to 1960, the world growth rate doubled from one to two percent a year. The starkness of this shift is better appreciated when cast against the growth rate of the 1800s, only three-tenths of one percent; a rate that did not reach nine-tenths of one percent until the early 1900s.

The portentousness of the population explosion is more dramatic when measured by the sheer number of people on the earth. According to demographers, in year one, A.D., the world population had reached only 250 million. It took 1650 years to double and until 1850 to reach the billion mark. The next doubling, however, to two billion, took only eighty years. From 1930 to 1960, the human count raced past the three billion mark. The next billion, bringing the total to four billion, was not expected to occur until 1980. The estimate proved overly modest, as every population estimate in the twentieth century has. By 1980, nearly 4.5 billion people existed on the planet. The best projections today are that more than a billion additional people per decade will be added, skyrocketing the world population to nearly 6.5 billion by the year 2000.

While the total numbers still climb perilously, primarily because of the preponderance in numbers of people in the child-bearing years, something totally unexpected is now happening. A glimmer of light flickers amidst the dark predictions. To the astonishment of population watchers, the rate of population growth has begun to decline, ever so slightly, on a worldwide average from the 2.1 percent peak in the 1970s to 1.78 percent in 1980. But the Catch-22 in that trend is that the growth rate is so disproportionate: the less developed regions will account for nine-tenths of the increase in world population during the next twenty years, the areas least able to bear it.

There is disagreement on what factors have slowed down the world growth rate. One camp emphasizes the widespread, although uneven, dissemination of contraceptives and family planning education. The other camp accredits the shift to a combination of those forces along with industrial development, a well-documented influence in lowering family size. Clearly, however, the process that has worked most effectively has been tying strong population-control programs (*à la* the Republic of China) to improved economic conditions.

For the population doomsayers and humanists who saw birth control as the key weapon against intractable population growth, the negative stance of the Vatican in the encyclical *Casti Canubii* was seen as an obdurate and irrelevant response to a *new* problem. The old moral view of birth control no longer applied in an overcrowded, half-starved world. Increasingly, it seemed there were compelling new reasons to employ birth control for social good.

Late in 1955, the moment of decision had come. Was he willing to be midwife to the birth of a new era in birth control, to attend the delivery of a tiny pill capable not only of taming the whirlwind of population growth, but of unfettering human sexuality? It was an immeasurably profound step, an historic benchmark of unparalleled significance. And one from which there would be no retreat. Rock had to be sure in his soul as well as his mind that the good of society was being served. In thinking it through, his reverence for marital love, for the paramount importance of the family and for women, married or single, who bore the brunt of repeated pregnancies, prevailed. Rock's basic concern for the well-being of the individual family had not really changed. It had enlarged. He now was convinced that control of "overfecundity" was necessary if the family of Man were to be preserved.

Still, he took his time and moved with thoughtful caution through every step in the testing of the new progestins. There were repeated conferences in Puerto Rico, Brookline, and Worcester. They checked and rechecked not only their own data, but some tentative trials with the Syntex pill carried out by Dr. Edward Tyler in Los Angeles. They culled analyses being made simultaneously by Searle's clinical staff. Rock leaned on Pincus for critical statistical data that showed which of the two finalist progestins — Searle's or Syntex's — had fewer side effects. Rock also reviewed with Garcia the medical findings, blood and reproductive tissue samples from the volunteers.

Before field trials could start, the critical decision had to be made on which pill was best. In the last analysis Rock relied on his own experienced instinct. He picked Searle's SC-4642 as "the pill of choice." "There was a mutual discussion about the choice. Rock's main concern was to set the thing up so that it would be to the patient's advantage, so the patient would profit by it and the patient would be protected. These are the things that Rock addressed himself to; the sort of things I addressed myself to. Pincus would figure out the statistics and the probabilities when there were dosage variations and so forth," Garcia recalled. It was time to go forward with the pill.

8

THE PILL IS APPROVED

ON all counts, Puerto Rico in 1956 was a perfect miniature world in which to test the pill. An island with limited land space, it already was feeling the crush of overpopulation. Moreover, in that period, its people were stationary, with little opportunity to move elsewhere. The island's poor economy was reflected in severe unemployment, abject housing, and low education. If the pill could work here, it could work anywhere.

A number of other sites were considered and rejected. Providence, Rhode Island, New York City, Japan, and Mexico. Massachusetts, of course, was excluded because of its laws that made birth control a felony. Puerto Rico remained the best bet. Ironically, because it was an intensely Catholic country no need was seen for anti–birth control laws in Puerto Rico and so none existed. It also offered another great advantage in that the Planned Parenthood movement had a well-established base in San Juan. Dr. Edris Rice-Wray, an impassioned believer in birth control, held a dual appointment as director of the U.S. Public Health Field Training Center associated with the university there and as medical director of the Puerto Rico Family Planning Association. She could be counted on to help in every way.

To get the first field trial started in April 1956, she suggested locating it in a huge new public housing development in Rio Piedras, a suburb of San Juan. Nearly all the families there had lived in hovels before coming to these public housing projects, *parcellas,* that the government erected. "Once they got into these very nice, comfortable quarters, they weren't anxious to move out again. The accommodations were virtually rent free and in some instances," Garcia explained, "their rent was put into an eventual ownership kind of arrangement." With better housing, the women wanted to improve other aspects of family life. Further, the superintendent of the housing project was a birth control aficionado, a former social worker for the housing project, a person familiar to the tenants, and was available to recruit volunteers.

As the trials began, an unexpected but fortuitous hitch developed. In one batch of the Enovid, the trade name for Searle's SC-4642, a minuscule amount of estrogen (actually a synthetic estrogen, mestranol) "contaminated" the lot. Production was revamped and the estrogen removed. To everyone's surprise, the pure progestin did not work as well. Women found they experienced a higher incidence of undesirable, breakthrough bleeding intermittently during the menstrual cycle, rather than at the end. Then, chemical analyses revealed that traces of mestranol had been present all the while in the original, effective lots of norethynodrel (Enovid). It was the unintended presence of synthetic estrogen that accounted for the better performance of the Searle product, rather than the Syntex version. The course of wisdom, obviously, was to deliberately retain some estrogen (mestranol) in the pill. Thereafter, small amounts of the companion hormone were designed into future batches in doses of 1.5 percent of the 10 milligram Enovid tablet.

To recruit the first set of one hundred volunteers, women who came to the Rio Piedras family planning clinic were asked if they would be interested in trying a new experimental birth control pill. Garcia can "still remember Rock asking the women whether they would be interested in something they could take as a pill each day that would prevent them from becoming pregnant. Their eyes would open up like saucers, and they would say, 'Why of course, why not?' There was always a very high recruitment no matter where we went, not only in Puerto Rico, but other parts of the world." Until that time, when they became desperate at becoming pregnant again, many of the Rio Piedras women underwent permanent sterilization by having their Fallopian tubes tied (tubal ligation). One sign of the acceptance of the pill was the drop in the tube-tying surgery.

The women's Catholicism did not prove to be a hurdle, as had been feared. "Among all Catholics there's a range of devotion from the fanatic to the devout, to the marginal," Garcia observed. "But the vast majority of the Catholics in Puerto Rico were just plain practical in their attitudes. They felt they had to choose between two evils. Maybe that wasn't the way they expressed it, but in their own way they were saying they had to choose between the evil of birth control and the evil of not being able to feed that extra mouth. The only point of religious contention was that they would rationalize that tubal ligation was a one-time sin. Once it was done, nothing could undo it. They could go to confession, receive forgiveness and be done with it. With the pill, the difficulty was they had to rationalize how they could live with a daily reminder that they were continuously preventing pregnancy, and therefore, in the Church's eyes, were in a chronic state of sinfulness. They overcame this by temporizing to the effect that the pill was a birth control technique they could reverse — unlike permanent steril- ization. They came around to the idea they were refraining from ovulation, instead of from sexual intercourse.

"Acceptance of that kind of thinking became very frightening to the hierarchy of the Catholic Church there. Despite admonitions by Cath- olic social workers, warnings from the pulpit, and outright condemna- tion over TV and in the Catholic press, the women just decided that the worst thing they could do was bring another baby into the world that they couldn't afford. They feared they might come to hate the child. To develop family problems was the greatest evil. For a while, when the women went to confession, if the priest noticed they hadn't been pregnant for a while, he'd openly ask them, 'Are you on the pill?' On the *damn* pill was the way it was actually phrased. Then, the Cath- olic Social Workers Guild put on a TV program and made a lot of statements about how dangerous the pill was. About 10 percent of the volunteers dropped out. All, *all* immediately became pregnant. After that we never had a problem enlisting volunteers. They came flocking, not just the indigent population, but schoolteachers, the social workers themselves, everybody," Garcia said. It was no joke for the impover- ished Puerto Rican women in the study. As the months went by and they did not get pregnant, they experienced the first freedom from preg- nancy they'd ever known. They were elated. Word spread by word-of- mouth week by week. Any need for recruitment vanished. The num- bers of women who came to the clinic, asking for the pill, mushroomed.

At Rock's and Garcia's insistence, each woman in the field trial re- ceived a full gynecological exam, including a Papanicolaou smear for detection of pre-cancerous changes in the tissue of the cervix. Any abnormalities were treated free of charge. For nearly all of the women, this sort of gynecological attention was totally new. They had been accustomed to seeing a doctor or a midwife only when they were giving birth. Anne Merrill, who had worked with Chang on the original animal studies with progestin at the Worcester Foundation, had come down to help with the Rio Piedras project. At first, she found it hard to accept that the women were interested in birth control. They looked like grandmothers, she noted, "all wizened and gaunt." Then she would find them to be only thirty to thirty-five years old, but already the mother of ten or more children plus innumerable miscarriages.

For Rock, Garcia, and Pincus, however, there remained additional factors of crucial importance to be investigated. Prior to Puerto Rico the pill had been given for relatively short periods of time, never longer than a half-dozen cycles. Even the dosage was a "best-guesstimate," the governing criterion that enough be given to assure freedom from pregnancy. The one thing that would scuttle the field trial was if any of the women became pregnant. That would undermine all confidence in the pill. The first dosage was 10 milligrams (1/2800 of an ounce).* But, at that dosage for prolonged periods, there were some questions that only sustained usage could answer. Its immediate safety was not the major worry. Rock was confident the pill per se was safe on a short-term basis because he had given far larger doses of the pill — up to 300 milligrams — to his original "Rock rebound" patients. The new questions turned on whether the constant use of the pill would alter the normal 50-50 ratio of boy-to-girl babies when the women would stop taking the progestin to become pregnant by choice; whether any permanent loss of fertility would result when the reproductive system was "banked" down for months to years; and whether any birth defects would ensue. There was indescribable relief and joy when subsequent pregnancies occurred within four months in 85 percent of the women who stopped the pill in order to get pregnant, when boys and girls arrived in the normal complement, and when no birth defects afflicted any of the infants.

Each of the women was warned that she might experience side effects such as transient nausea, headaches, or slight weight gains during the first few months of pill use. Most of the women didn't mind. Such discomforts were minor, they felt, compared to the alternative — another pregnancy every year. Nonetheless the question of side effects had to be dealt with. In Dr. Rice-Wray's group, some 17 percent of

---

* Later, lower doses of 5 and 2.5 milligrams also were tested.

the women experienced "unpleasant" side effects to a noticeable degree. This may have been due to her persistent inquiries about side effects, which, psychologically, could have "suggested" the idea of nausea and discomfort to the women. Underlying guilt over practicing birth control may also have been a factor. At any rate, Rice-Wray's first summary report concluded that the pill "causes too many side-reactions to be acceptable generally."

Pincus, armed with his previous research experience with Hoagland on psychological manifestations, designed tests to probe further into the suggestability factor. Placebos were given to a group of women who were protected from pregnancy by other means. Their experience was cast against a group of women given the genuine pill. Pincus found that the placebo group "suffered" the same 17 percent incidence of side effects as the pill takers. In another group given genuine pills, but no warning of side effects, only 7 percent complained of them.

Insofar as contraception was concerned, the studies exceeded their wildest dreams. At the end of the first nine months of field tests, some forty-seven woman-years of experience with the pill had been clocked. Not a single woman suffered any dire consequences, and not one who took the pill as directed was pregnant.

Based on the first round of Puerto Rican contraception studies and a handful of small ancillary trials in the U.S. where the progestins were given for therapeutic reasons, the Food and Drug Administration approved Enovid — but only as a *treatment* for menstrual disorders. It was nonetheless a major first step toward full licensure as a birth control pill. Mrs. McCormick, who only months earlier had impatiently observed that "everything [is going] as slow as molasses," now exulted over the FDA approval. With typical canniness she understood what the limited licensure really meant. She wrote: "Of course this use of the oral contraceptive for menstrual disorders is leading inevitably to its use against pregnancy — and to me — this stepping stone of gradual approach to the pregnancy problem via the menstrual one is a very happy and fortunate course of procedure."

Although Mrs. McCormick then could see how well the work was proceeding, she realized it would take much more to bring the trials to complete fruition. She treasured Pincus's scientific acumen, but she knew that Rock was the key. She wrote: "Pincus cannot do any more experiments with patients [a reference to the Worcester Hospital episode] . . . he is not a clinician and is not as reliable in examinations as is Rock, who, you know, has a perfectionist standard from which he will not deviate nor rely on anyone else! Rock's work should be expanded. He is unique for us at present. . . ." Other people's part in the work, she observed in 1956, was all well and good, but "it can't take the place of Rock's. Indeed, nothing I know can." Another time she wrote: "We can trust his data."

Neither Rock, Pincus, nor Garcia felt the Rio Piedras studies were sufficient. More experience was needed before any attempt could be made to go after FDA approval of Enovid as an out-and-out birth control pill. A second Puerto Rican trial was quickly set up in the village of Humacoa. Once again the choice was made, in part, because a woman doctor who was enthusiastic about birth control was already on the scene. At Humacoa, under more primitive and often taxing conditions, the medical missionary Dr. Adeline Pendleton Satterthwaite duplicated the trial procedures initiated by Dr. Rice-Wray. After the first nine months of the trial, Dr. Rice-Wray had been fired from her government post as a public health worker. At the same time the number of women in her Rio Piedras study nearly doubled. And soon after that, a third field trial was established in Haiti at the invitation of the island's ruler, "Papa Doc" Duvalier.

Suddenly, testing was no longer the main issue. Public acceptance was. No matter how well the pill worked, the entire endeavor would degenerate into an exercise in futility if the public opposed the pill. The Rio Piedras venture had proved that those pregnancy-beset women wanted the pill desperately. On the other hand the trial had generated a lot of heat not only from the Catholic Church there, but government officials as well. Even though Searle officials had okayed supplying Enovid for the field trials, knowing the purpose was to test the pill's contraceptive use, the company originally had viewed progestin primarily as a marketable treatment for menstrual problems. Syntex (having no marketing capabilities) had licensed Djerassi's progestin, labeled Norlutin, to the Parke-Davis pharmaceutical company to be marketed for the same good, but limited, purpose.

However, as the field trials unequivocally demonstrated the overriding contraceptive effect of the pill, Searle officials became wracked with worry about the possibility of a severe public backlash over the "immorality" of such a birth control agent. They feared it would ruin the company. G. D. Searle Company had been founded in the late 1800s by an Indian pharmacist, Gideon Searle. From the start the firm had an enviable, ethical reputation. What terrified its officers in 1958 was the prospect of public condemnation for going into the birth control business. It was a tantalizing dilemma. On one side was a potential new product gold mine that seemingly would never run out: the sale of millions of pills to succeeding generations of women. On the other lay possible ruin, if the company were blacklisted for dealing in an unsavory business. After all, Goodyear Rubber never publicized its condom business, even though the sale of all brands of condoms in the U.S. in 1958 was a $150 million annual market. The federal and state governments in 1959 still wouldn't provide a penny for family planning for the poor at home or abroad, under any circumstances. Diaphragms were still obtained almost secretly by middle- and upper-class women. Contraception, despite Mrs. Sanger's steadily advancing birth control movement, still depended largely upon word-of-mouth indoctrination.

In a special report on the pill carried in *Fortune* magazine in April 1958, the good and bad connotations were juxtapositioned. "The promise is an inspiring one to those who believe in birth control as a means to a healthier society and to Neo-Malthusians who see it as a solution to the world-wide problems of overpopulation. [But to] descend from the moral to the material, there may well be some businessmen and economists who would wonder whether it was good for the *economy* to introduce anything that would depress the birth rate, at least of Americans." Lots of new babies "sold" a lot of goods — baby food, baby clothes, baby furnishings, baby appliances, and even a lot of home expansion and houses. Furthermore, they kept mothers at home buying an inexhaustible number of household products.

On the surface, the post–World War II societal pattern still held sway. Well into the 1950s America continued to revel in an unparalleled baby boom, one that exceeded its counterpart anywhere in Europe and persisted much longer. In the U.S., children were said to be "cheaper by the dozen." Mothering was big business in the postwar economy. With great zest, women turned away from the job opportunities ushered in by the wartime manpower shortage and reembraced the *Kinder, Küche, Kirche* model of earlier generations, sloganized by Hitler's Third Reich. The traditional, large, old-time family seemingly would persevere forever.

Everyone was in for the surprise of the century. Beneath the surface, a strange restlessness that was at first barely perceptible was beginning to stir. Families were mobile as never before. Changing job markets uprooted young families again and again. They were hemmed into small houses, cramped by rising costs. Husbands and wives found themselves trapped economically and emotionally by large families in a new era when grandparents were no longer near at hand to help out and domestic help was neither available, affordable, nor democratic. "It was a strange stirring, a sense of dissatisfaction," Betty Friedan later called it in her book *The Feminine Mystique* in 1963. "Each suburban wife struggled with it alone. All they had to do was to devote their lives from earliest girlhood to finding a man and bearing children. Where once they had two children, they now had four, five, six. By the end of the fifties, the United States birthrate was overtaking India's." But they and their husbands were beginning to ask, "Is this all there is?"

Yet, at the time that Searle's masterminds had to weigh the financially tempting but potentially ruinous decision whether to openly introduce a birth control pill, the flickering new interest in family limitation was not yet apparent. At Searle, however, the pill had two unexpected champions, John Searle himself and Dr. Irwin C. Winter (I.C. or Icy Winter as he is known), the company's director of clinical research. According to Celso Garcia, "Most people are not aware of it, but the fact is that Jack Searle was genuinely interested in the population problem. He was very active in the population control movement and donated enormous amounts of money to it before he began making any money from the oral contraceptive." Winter, who in appearance, speech, and mannerisms remarkably resembles the homespun character-actor Edgar Buchanan, had a reason closer to home. "Two of my sisters were medical missionaries in India. My father was a minister in the Dutch Reformed Church, now Congregational. I was exposed early to world population problems and through my sisters I knew very personally about the terrible poverty, sickness, starvation and death caused by population growth in India. At the same time, I can't over-emphasize the restrictive atmosphere here [in the U.S.] over birth control. It was more than considerably difficult to do anything about it. Because Enovid prevented ovulation, it took a number of months to get the first FDA approval in 1957 for it as a prescriptive medicine for serious menstrual problems. Even that much came about in part because the medical director of the FDA was a friend of mine."

Winter, who had joined the Searle staff in 1946, first met Rock in connection with Rock's infertility work. "At any rate we got to know John Rock very well. He was a complete gynecologist. His patients thought he was wonderful. . . . I got him to treat some friends of mine who were having infertility problems. I liked him very much and we became very good friends. He taught me how to smoke a pipe without having it go out; you just blow through it once in a while." Winter also knew Pincus. "It was actually Pincus and Al Raymond [Searle's director of research] who decided in the late 1940s that Searle should get into the steroid business. When Pincus first became interested in developing contraceptives, he had an idea for developing a preparation (anti-hyaluronidase) that would block the enzyme that activates sperm, thereby allowing sperm to penetrate the egg. [This idea was based on Chang's capacitation work.] Pincus had some success with rabbits using it. We gave it a try. The study fell through, though. It just became too complicated. Then, later Pincus became interested in the progestational substances and we sent him a whole series of them. Pincus had become very ardent by that time in his search for contraceptives. Rock was too. He was very genuinely concerned about overpopulation and the need for safe and effective means of birth control. There's no question about it."

Winter also verifies that it was Rock who made the final selection of the Searle product. "Rock picked it. He and Pincus met together constantly and discussed all the problems. But Rock picked it. Nowadays, Syntex [and Djerassi] make a big thing of the claim that they were the real discoverers of the first oral contraceptive substance. And in the sense that Djerassi patented the first one, that's correct. But they didn't do a thing with it beyond its use as a drug for menstrual problems. Parke-Davis wasn't interested in getting into the birth control game. You must understand that social attitudes were a big issue. A birth control pill had to overcome serious public attitudes that questioned whether such a thing was moral, ethical, or good. Many of the pharmaceutical manufacturers felt this was not a suitable business for an ethical drug house. In fact, the then president of Parke-Davis, a good friend of John Searle's, called him and told him he was crazy to even think of doing such a thing. Life was a bit different then. The young people don't realize . . . they don't know anything about how it was. You remember right through the Eisenhower administration, he said, no federal money will *ever* be used for birth control programs."

Parke-Davis went beyond warning Searle that a birth control pill was "crazy" business. Parke-Davis made it company policy to stay out of the contraceptive field. The company, based in the intensely Catholic diocese of Detroit, issued unequivocating statements to the *Detroit Free Press* that the pill was not in the company's plans. "Its policy is to keep out of the contraceptive field, and it will never recommend, nor even test, Norlutin for contraceptive purposes — only as a therapeutic agent for disorders of the female reproductive system," one report proclaimed. Even after the pill won FDA licensure as a contraceptive, Parke-Davis refused to turn over the monkey studies it had conducted on the pill to Syntex so the findings could be used to substantiate Norlutin's efficacy as a contraceptive. Syntex had turned to the Ortho Division of Johnson & Johnson to market Norlutin. As a result, it was 1962 before Ortho could get Syntex's version of the pill, now rechristened Ortho-Novum, on the market. For two years Searle had an exclusive birth control pill product line. In *The Politics of Contraception,* Djerassi's frustration is still evident: "Parke-Davis's apprehension about a possible boycott of its other products as a result of a potential Catholic backlash was perhaps not unreasonable, but such a consumer backlash never developed." Djerassi implies that Syntex's offer of marketing rights to Parke-Davis was an almost altruistic move, "a way of making up" for earlier misunderstandings between Syntex's founder, Russell Marker, and Parke-Davis. But he seemingly contradicts himself when he also points out that three years earlier Syntex had extended the option to Charles Pfizer and Co. — "but Pfizer had not exercised it because its president, who was a very active Roman Catholic lay person, felt that Pfizer should not touch any agent even potentially related to birth control." The upshot of the whole thing was that Syntex had to "start almost from scratch to find another marketing candidate" after Parke-Davis refused to touch a birth control pill. "In 1964, Parke-Davis finally woke up to the facts of life," Djerassi wrote, "and decided to enter the contraceptive market after all."

To Searle's credit, the company stayed in the game in the face of great odds — or so they thought. They contributed the pills used in the Puerto Rico trials, "on a gamble." There was no denying that the pill represented a bonanza of unimaginable proportions. The pill could be sold to millions of women possibly throughout their thirty childbearing years. Potentially each one of them would take 240 tablets a year. (The original price was fifty-five cents each, or about eleven dollars a month, though mass production would bring that price down. Today, the pill is sold in bulk to international family planning organizations for use in developing countries for seventeen cents for a month's supply.)

Before the final decision to "go all the way" with the pill was made, Searle's public relations mentor, James W. Irwin, decided to at least test the water of public opinion. He planted two major articles about the pill in the *Saturday Evening Post* and a third one in *Reader's Digest*. The magazines' editors were warned, up front, that Searle felt the subject was dynamite, sensitive and controversial. The magazines had to risk alienating their readers. The articles ran, carrying the news that the pill, the very one that was solving menstrual disorders, also looked like a perfect birth control agent, and that it was being tested for that purpose in Puerto Rico. Then, everyone waited. And absolutely nothing happened. There was no adverse reaction whatsoever to the stories. Later, Searle analyzed their own needless fears and concluded that women taking Enovid for menstrual disorders had begun to spread the word about the sexual freedom that its use also conferred.

The great selling point was that the pill separated any act of contraception from the sex act. "I know one couple who, in the pre-pill days, had three extra children," Winter said, "because the wife said very frankly, on cold winter nights she hated to get out of their warm bed and go on the cold floor in her bare feet to the bathroom to insert her diaphragm. You know, those are the realities." With the pill, women found they could take it and forget about it. Women who had become paranoid with fear of another pregnancy and resisted the sexual advances of their husbands were suddenly once again willing, enthusiastic sex partners. Sex got back its highly pleasurable spontaneity. Before going to bed there was no need to plan ahead. Nice "ladies," many of whom used diaphragms but found the process repugnant — the squatting down, inserting and removing them — or husbands who had to have a condom handy even though they found them sensually restrictive, discovered the true joy of unrestrained sex. It seemed almost too good to be true. Sex was set free not only from pregnancy but from advance preparation.

Searle geared up for mass production. It was an act of rare industrial courage. *Fortune* magazine had touted its audience off the idea in 1958: There is a vast difference between dispensing the drug as a safe means of inducing temporary sterility for therapeutic purposes and dispensing it for "habitual use" as a standard contraceptive. "It will take perhaps five years of research to satisfy any drug firm that is ready to apply to the Food and Drug Administration for permission to so label its product; and it would take five years after that before the FDA — which says it may well require clinical data on 'thousands' of women not 500 — would approve such application." What the editors of *Fortune* did not realize was that nearly a thousand women in Puerto Rico already were enrolled in trials. Together, they were clocking a total of fifteen thousand cycles of experience with the pill. Besides that, some of the Puerto Rican volunteers — the original medical students — had been using the pill steadily for nearly six years. No medicine in history up to that time had undergone as extensive a trial run. The evidence was largely in.

Beyond that, by late 1959, another half-million American women were taking the same pill — either as Enovid or Norlutin — for treatment of their menstrual disorders. It was *amazing* that so many women suddenly had menstrual disorders requiring treatment with the pill, women who had never seemed to have menstrual problems before. I.C. Winter understood why. The FDA license mandated that the drug carry a warning to doctors that women would not ovulate while taking it. "It was like a free ad," Winter wryly noted. Very quickly, doctors who had theretofore been less than sympathetic about marginal menstrual disorders found it very advantageous to prescribe the pill to treat them. Catholic doctors similarly became more than willing to help their patients "regulate" their cycles; the better to practice "rhythm," of course, later on. Meanwhile, the women had a vacation from fears of pregnancy. The same doctors, who had never tolerated any mention of sexual matters, now became very amenable to bringing the subject up. The same applied to their women patients. Both doctor and patient knew the pill's contraceptive power. Pincus helped matters along by announcing that the birth control pill was on the way every time he attended scientific meetings. The meetings were stopping points on a world trip undertaken with his wife, underwritten by undepletable funds of Mrs. McCormick.

Meanwhile, Rock was biding his time until the studies were complete. He had no doubts of the pill's efficacy and safety. His long years of using progesterones, and using them in high doses on his infertile women patients, had convinced him of the absence of any "serious" side effects. His and Garcia's meticulous medical monitoring of the women in the Puerto Rico trials reassured him. Not a single woman in those trials developed either blood clotting problems (later associated with pill use, most notably when combined with smoking) or any sign that the pill could induce cancerous tissue changes. To the contrary, Rock always believed that the pill would ultimately prove to be somewhat protective against cancer — as it now appears to be. His surmise that this would be the case was largely instinctive, an outgrowth of his long-standing impression that women who had children suffered fewer reproductive organ cancers than the childless. During the 1960s, Dr.

Robert Kistner was the first to demonstrate at the Boston Hospital for Women (Lying-In Division) that the combination forms of the pill did exert some beneficial influence against pre-cancerous changes in vaginal and uterine tissue, though the effect was not great enough to serve as an anti-cancer treatment once the malignancy was established.

When the studies began to reach to ten thousand cycles on the pill, however, Rock was ready to take it into the public domain. He and Garcia, by that time, were satisfied it was safe *enough*. As Garcia summed it up: "All of the indications that we had were that there were either no side effects or none of any consequence. They were all over-exaggerated because of the general opposition to the idea of birth control. Attitudes change, but at that particular time, contraception was a dirty word in the households of most people in this country. It was something that you mentioned *sotto voce*. It's hard to put yourself back in the context of those times because most of us forget the unpleasant things about life. That's fortunate for the human being, but unfortunate for the historian. There is still, and was then, far less concern about women's incredible burden. It's not easy to go through nine months of pregnancy. Any sort of physiological deficit may mean her life. It's one hell of an imposition to put on anybody. But no one showed the same concern for poor pregnant women that they showed over the 'hazards' the pill would subject them to."

Early in 1959, all the key participants — Searle, Rock, Garcia, and Pincus — were agreed that the time had come to beard the lions of the FDA in their den. Searle, now, was pressing them to "hurry" with the test results. Pincus saw no reason to test the pill endlessly to appease "the qualms of officialdom." Rock and Garcia, who had personally checked every patient record — and had overseen the checking of each patient, individually — were prepared to defend the pill's harmlessness when properly used under a physician's supervision. I. C. Winter, who also bird-dogged every medical report from the field trials, concurred. He neither wanted to risk harm to the millions of women whom he was confident would want to use it, nor have the drug boomerang on Searle. Searle was going out on the longest limb in pharmaceutical history in backing it. "Searle was the only company with the guts to do it," Garcia pointed out.

Searle filed its application to license the pill as a contraceptive on October 29, 1959. The first series of cases upon which the application was based reported the experience of 897 women, representing 801.6 woman-years and 10,427 cycles. At that time the FDA was empowered

only to require that a drug be "safe": Not until the 1962 Kefauver-
Harris amendments to the Federal Food Drug and Cosmetic Act did
the FDA's jurisdiction legally encompass a drug's effectiveness and reliability. Countless drugs were approved on the flimsiest of evidence.
The real emphasis of the FDA at the time was on quality control in
the purity of manufacturing of any new drug. Whether it worked as
claimed was secondary, and safety was a very relative matter. When
for its own reasons, however, the FDA wanted to delay approval of a
new drug, even back then, it had tactics for doing so. For example, if
the FDA did not take action on a new drug application within ninety
days or sooner, the agency could notify the applicant the bid was being
extended for an additional six months. With the pill, the extension ploy
was used twice.

"I remember it vividly," recalled Winter. "The FDA was using as a
part-time reviewer a practicing obstetrician-gynecologist, Dr. Pasquale
DeFelice from Georgetown Medical Center. He was a relatively young
man and obviously a Catholic. He went over the material submitted
and later we got a very long letter, not very coherently expressed, stat-
ing why the FDA couldn't approve Enovid as an oral contraceptive."
DeFelice was thirty-five years old, a graduate of Fordham University,
a Jesuit school, and Georgetown Medical School in Washington, D.C.,
another Catholic-oriented institution. Although he'd completed his
training and was qualified in obstetrics and gynecology, he was not yet
board certified. DeFelice had joined the FDA staff in 1956 and was
well aware that, in some instances, "someone would submit an application for sterile water in the treatment of arthritis and if you couldn't
prove that it *didn't* work — rather than that it *did* — it would get approved. But we tried harder than people think to use the extension
clause as a gimmick to make the drug companies provide more information, when we got some of those ridiculous applications.

"When a new drug application came in for the birth control pills, it
was — needless to say — revolutionary for that indication! It was a
whole new bag of beans. Everything else up to that time was a drug to
treat a diseased condition. Here, suddenly, was a pill to be used to treat
a healthy person and for long-term use. We really went overboard.
Even though the pill had been through more elaborate testing than any
drug in the FDA's history, there was a lot of opposition. Everyone was
afraid of the pill. No other pill ever was put through anything like the
tests for '*the* pill.' Penicillin went through the FDA process very easily
even though five hundred people a year still die from penicillin reac-

tions. With the pill, however, the FDA had to come out of the licensing absolutely clean! We got all the studies, every page of them, from the projects in Puerto Rico and Haiti. Some of the women had been using the pill for as long as five years and there just were no significant side effects. But we were in no hurry to put the FDA stamp of approval on it."

There was only one way to handle it, only one person who could do it. Rock, himself, would have to confront the objectors at the FDA. "We asked for a hearing and asked John to come along," said I. C. Winter. (Dr. J. William Crosson, Searle's assistant medical director, went too.) At that time DeFelice's office was in a barrackslike temporary wooden building that had been put up during the First World War. The hearing was held on a bitterly cold day late in December 1950. Winter also recalled that "we had to stand in a barren little entryway for more than an hour and a half until DeFelice showed up. I felt at the time that we were left waiting to discourage us. There wasn't even a chair to sit down on. There is no question, the long, cold wait was hard on Rock. Though he was in great shape and an imposing figure, he was seventy years old at the time. Once we were inside, however, Rock carried out the whole thing. It was quite an impassioned discussion."

DeFelice, according to Winter, brought up associations between the use of steroids and cancer "and about everything else imaginable." Rock, towering above DeFelice, kept referring to him as "young man." Rock responded to the cancer allegations by saying, "I don't know how much training *you've* had in *female cancer, young man,* but I've had considerable!" DeFelice next contended that there hadn't been enough use of the pill up to that point, so it couldn't be considered proven. Rock rallied back, "If your garage is on fire, you do not wait to see if your bucket has a hole in it before trying to throw water on the blaze." He was, of course, referring to the population dilemma. "Then," Winter recalled, "DeFelice brought up moral and religious objections — saying the Catholic Church would never approve of it. I can still see Rock standing there, his face composed, his eyes riveted on DeFelice and then in a voice that would congeal your soul, he said, 'Young man, don't you sell *my* Church short!' "

That was the end of the hearing, or so DeFelice thought. He told Rock, Winter, and Crossen, he would send the data to outside consultants and referees. Rock was annoyed at best because so young and inexperienced a doctor was assigned to such a monumentally important matter. "In came a nondescript, thirty-year-old from Washington. Can you imagine, the FDA gave *him* the job of deciding. I was furious," Rock said. "In effect, this young man had said to us, 'Very glad to have talked with you. I'll go over it all again and you'll hear from me.' I stood up and I grabbed him by his jacket lapels and I said, 'No, you won't take it all home with you. You'll decide right now.' He said, 'Oh, all right.' I don't think he knew the significance of what he was doing."

DeFelice's memory of the occasion is not precisely the same. "You have to remember, there I was, a thirty-five-year-old qualified but not yet board-certified OB-GYN man. Standing before me was John Rock, *the light of the obstetrical world!* Yes, there was *some* discussion of the morals of the pill, what was going to happen if it was approved. But I personally was not concerned about the morality of it. I don't remember taking an adverse position on it. I think I told him [Rock], 'If Presbyterians and Baptists can use birth control pills and go to heaven, why can't Catholics.' I tell you very frankly, I'm a philosophical Catholic. At Fordham, I took a lot of philosophy. I felt the Church was really not right about birth control and I never could understand why the popes didn't back down on it. Rock was a gentleman about the whole thing. He called me on the phone several times. I had my job to look out for, you know what I mean. I think about Rock every now and then. He was a professional figure of great standing. Anything he said had to be listened to. I've only met about three doctors in my entire life who I would trust with anything. Rock was one of them. He still is.

"As much as I was impressed by Rock and the study data, we got Winter to promise to do lab tests on five hundred cases detailing any blood-clotting mechanisms. Very frankly, the tests showed no significant difference in the blood-clotting mechanisms. Nor did I expect them to. I really only asked for them because we know, empirically, that pregnant women tend to have a higher incidence of blood clots. Since the pill created a pseudo-pregnancy I thought we'd better double-check. They, the Searle people, were very anxious to get the pill on the market. The important things to us at the FDA were quality control, purity of product and side effects. Actually, Searle wanted us to license lower doses of Enovid right away, 5 and 2.5 milligram doses as well as the 10. But, it wasn't because they were worried about the side effects. It was because the 10 milligram pills cost them a lot of money. They were worried about costs.

"But I knew what was going to happen once we licensed it. I knew that birth control pills would be flying out the windows. Everybody and her sister would be taking it. You know something: I was stupid. I should be a millionaire. I should have bought Searle stock, but I didn't. Somehow I thought I shouldn't since I was the person who approved it. But I have often wondered why I never got an award for okaying the pill. It changed the whole economy of the United States."

Today, DeFelice, who now is head of the obstetrics-gynecology service at Morris Cafritz Memorial Hospital in a Washington, D.C., suburb, "has no qualms about putting women on the pill when everything else is unsatisfactory. With all the scare stories, some of my patients went back to condoms and diaphragms, but very few are satisfied with them. When used properly — not in women who smoke or women over forty — the pill is as safe as anything else. People don't bother to point out it has a lower risk than abortion or pregnancy. There are so many idiots in the United States, they keep harping on the pill's risk. But there are five hundred abortions a day in Washington, D.C., now. How about that risk?!" *

However convinced DeFelice was of the pill's safety and convenience, or how much he questions the Church's anti–birth control stance, he personally pursued his own course. He fathered ten children.

On April 22, 1960, DeFelice formally notified the Searle Co., in a letter directed to the attention of Crosson, that the supplemental information sought was received, along with a new supplemental application for licensure. The letter informed Searle that the approval of the pill was, as of that date, conditionally effective, and that full approval would come as soon as specimens of final labeling were submitted, in accordance with "draft copy," then in the hands of the FDA. It all became official — and public — the following month. The historic date was May 11, 1960.

In a summary of the background and reasons for the FDA's approval, William H. Kessenich, head of the New Drug Branch, wrote George P. Larrick, then FDA commissioner, that "because of the considerable general interest and possible objections from some quarters with respect to our action in clearing the drug for such use [contraception], we are furnishing the following information concerning the basis for our action."

After noting specific data, the letter pointed out that "any objection by the patient to the side effects, of course, would result in voluntary

---

* The risk from properly performed abortions is exceedingly small — only one death in 100,000.

discontinuance of the use of the product and therefore are of no serious concern." In response to conjecture that the pill would leave some women permanently sterile, the letter also noted "that 83 percent of those not using other contraceptives became pregnant . . . six months after discontinuing use of the drug. Dr. Rock did follicle counts on the ovary to be sure that the potential for production of the egg was left intact on 15 women taking Enovid for 2–20 months and found no change from normal controls." But most revealing was the disclosure that the FDA had queried sixty-one professors of obstetrics and gynecology at medical schools around the country about whether the pill should be licensed for birth control. "We were pleased to receive a 100 percent response. The answers we received were as follows: 14 of the professors felt they did not have sufficient data to reach a conclusion; 26 said yes, it should be allowed for contraceptive purposes; 21 of the professors said that even though they could give no specific reason for reaching this conclusion, they must say no; however, 2 of the no's were based on religious grounds and others may have been." Another summary, prepared by Deputy FDA Commissioner John L. Harvey, further noted, "Although we recognize the presence of moral issues, they do not come within the jurisdiction of the Food and Drug Administration."

The last word, rightfully, was to be Katherine Dexter McCormick's. Referring to a lecture on the pill given at Harvard's Biological Laboratories, she wrote Mrs. Sanger: "They have been working for years on *basic research* of the human reproductive system — all for sound knowledge and learning doubtless, but for practical aid *nothing* — and the abortions merrily went on before their very eyes! Personally I doubt if *they*, at Harvard, would ever have found an oral contraceptive!"

9

A NEW QUESTION CONFRONTS THE CHURCH

THE pill was different: totally, uniquely, undeniably, unmistakably different.

For the Roman Catholic Church, the last great bastion of opposition to any form of birth control — except periodic or prolonged sexual abstinence — the pill was a particular bedevilment. It posed a different contraceptive idea than any that Church thinkers had ever before had to contemplate.

Church authorities soon realized that the pill's champion, John Rock, was different, too; far different than anyone else in modern times to confront them publicly on such an important moral issue. Both the pill and Rock caught the Church off-balance on its most tenuous doctrinal ground: its superficial grasp of the profound role of human sexuality in personality formation and thereafter, as the most pervasive, intimate and enduring aspect of adult life.

The pill also brought to the fore the Church's vacillating view of woman's role in the whole matter of sex and motherhood. In one guise she was still the eternal temptress Eve, the cause of the spiritual downfall of the human race; and in the other, the exalted embodiment of motherhood, the giver and nurturer of new life.

Rock's knowledge of the entire human reproductive experience far exceeded that of the ecclesiastics'. Between the two, Rock and the pill, his *damn pill* as some called it, the Church was suddenly forced to reexamine its fundamental position on birth control and, further, to do so in the full glare of world attention.

The most difficult point to deal with was that the pill wasn't an "artificial" form of birth control in the sense that Church Fathers had become accustomed to thinking about contraception. It wasn't mechanistic. It didn't kill or spill or block the passage of sperm the way all previous methods of "artificial" birth control had. The pill did not act in any way against the male seed, the historically protected male factor. Thus, it was outside the classic prohibitions so indelibly ingrained in nearly all religious guidelines on contraception, not just the Catholic rules.

While it is familiarly thought that Western religious bans on birth control are relatively new — only a century or two old — the genesis of anti–birth control thinking for Christians dates back to the first centuries after Christ's death. Its roots lie in an anti-marriage, anti-procreation movement that grew out of the idea that because Christ had come and redeemed mankind there no longer was any need for future generations to be born. Since Heaven awaited everyone alive, why perpetuate an earthbound existence? Within various sects of Christians, called Gnostics, two lines of behavior were embraced. Those on the left cast off all previous stoic Judaic teachings and indulged in unbridled sexual wantonness, but excluded childbearing and marriage. Those on the right were strict ascetics, decrying all forms of physical pleasure — excluding sex, marriage, and consequent childbearing from their lives. In "this seething Alexandrian world, within the Christian community, marriage was scorned as sinful or as useless," as John Noonan put it in his *Contraception: A History of Its Treatment by Theologians and Canonists.* In response to both extremes, it fell to Clement of Alexandria, in the second century, to be the first Christian theologian who was forced to confront in a Christian light the question of what was the meaning of marriage. (Nearly two thousand years later, the pertinence of that question was still alive to be confronted anew by the Ecumenical Council, Vatican II.) Clement's answer was direct: the purpose of marriage was procreation. He declared that the Christian law is for "husbands to use their wives moderately and only for the raising up of children. . . . To have coition other than to procreate children is to do injury to nature." This rationale, vital to the survival of Christianity in the era in which it arose, formed the underpinnings upon which the Catholic Church still largely builds its case.

Over the centuries, Western religious instruction regarding birth control has moved along a sliding scale of acceptance. While birth control was not generally sanctioned by Protestantism until the early 1930s, today, nearly all Protestant churches — with the exception of some conservative fundamentalist groups — approve the full range of modern contraceptive methods available to both men and women. In the Judaic tradition, any immorality ascribed to contraception was and is wholly male and sperm-centered. The husband may not do anything physically or use any device that interferes with the transmission of the seed of life, but no contraceptive limitations are placed on his wife. Only within the official Catholic stance is the prohibition still absolute against all "artificial" forms of birth control.

The Catholic viewpoint also embodied the old theological idea that artificial forms of contraception are "homicidal," in the sense that the male seed is "killed" before it has a chance to carry out its God-given purpose — procreation. A woman's use of a diaphragm, douche, or spermicidal jelly or a man's use of a condom or his practice of premature withdrawal then amounts to a form of murder. "So many conceptions prevented, so many homicides" is an often-repeated admonition in authoritative teachings of the Church. Although that reasoning is not frequently expressed today, until a generation ago it was employed interchangeably by Catholics against both birth control and abortion. Just as abortion is held to be the taking of a newly conceived life, "artificial" birth control was said to be the taking of an intended life. Preservation of the egg and sperm during the life-*giving* process was seen as but a short step away from protection of an embryo or fetus from abortion.

This line of reasoning also bolstered the Church's ill-defined view of sex as a necessary evil. Sex outside of marriage was, of course, always forbidden, and even within marriage it was to be practiced judiciously: to relieve male concupiscence and to produce children. Sex that was protected against pregnancy was tantamount to frustrating the Lord's will.

The most dominant vein of Christian thinking on contraception, however, derives from the thirteenth-century teachings of St. Thomas Aquinas on "natural law." In simplified terms, contraception is regarded as a "sin against nature" because the sex organs, according to the Divine Plan, were instituted for the *inseminating* function. They were intended as generative organs, exclusively. Any other use was sinful. That reasoning accounted for why masturbation was wrong, along with homosexuality, bestiality, and "unnatural" positions of the sex act. The "fit way" for performing the sex act was with the woman beneath the man. This reflected both the natural superiority of man over woman and also further protected the male seed. Should the woman lie above the man, the seed might spill out. Modern Catholic theologians stress that the Thomistic argument centered squarely on the male *inseminating* aspect of sex relations.

The pill introduced a whole new dimension not only to the concept of contraception, but also to human sexuality. This was purely a woman's agent. The pill called into the open *her* role, *her* equal partnership in conception, and most of all, *her* personal, private, and total control over it. In fairness, the Roman Catholic Church was far from alone in its concern over sexual and marital morality. In most cultures, as the Redemptorist-theologian-sociologist Francis X. Murphy points out, sex has always had religious and ethical connotations: "Though many individuals and people today treat sex as a purely personal matter, the majority of mankind does acknowledge religious sanctions for human conduct and up to contemporary times most peoples considered conception and birth within the sphere of the sacred." * Back when the pill arrived, however, the Roman Catholic hierarchy stood virtually alone in its intense preoccupation with sex, even within marriage. Use of the pill amounted to a transcendent change in sexual power. For the first time, sexual freedom could be the same for women as it had always been for men. Other contraceptive methods involved preparations at the time of the sex act, including the immediate availability of contraceptive devices, water, and/or other substances. The very aspect of the pill that made it most appealing to married couples — its separation from the sex act — also made it "dangerous" morally. Taken privately at some point in the day, the pill protected women should spontaneous opportunities for sexual relations occur. If she chose, a woman could take the pill without anyone being the wiser — even her husband. Not only could she regulate her own fertility, but, in effect, his, too. And it was obvious that she could easily and freely indulge in sex relations with any man without fear that an unwanted pregnancy would reveal her clandestine activities. The prospects were utterly paralyzing in many quarters beyond religious. Summing up the resistance of those

---

* Murphy, *Catholic Perspectives on Population Issues* (Population Reference Bureau, 1975).

who opposed legalizing birth control, especially because of the pill, Massachusetts legislator William X. Wall exclaimed in horror: "No way should this be allowed. If she's gonna play, she's gonna pay!"

There was no question that the pill threw the issue of sex, as well as birth control, wide open for the Church. It didn't happen in a vacuum, however. Voices inside the Catholic Church as well as out in the world began to protest the repressive sexual constraints of the past. The idea that sexual *pleasure* within marriage was morally acceptable began to seep into religious thinking by the mid-1850s. Then, the French Jesuit John Gury in a Vatican-approved statement first held that sexual intercourse between spouses was lawful, among other reasons, to "foster or show mutual love." At the turn of the century, the German theologian John Becker vigorously defended pleasure as a *proper* purpose in marital intercourse. According to John T. Noonan in his exhaustive history of contraception (and its treatment by Catholic theologians): "It would be fair to describe the position as common after 1900. Pleasure as a purpose, then received guarded acceptance." Not until after World War I, however, did a Catholic professor of philosophy, Dietrich von Hildebrand, at the University of Munich, intertwine sex and love with marital fidelity. The *coup de grâce* on the meaning of sex in marriage, however, was delivered in 1935 by the German philosopher-zoologist-theologian-priest Hubert Doms. His position was that "in intimate love . . . the two partners give themselves in an act which contains the abandonment and enjoyment of the whole person and is not simply an isolated activity of [sexual] organs." Noonan states: "[Dom] said eloquently what serious Catholic laymen were waiting to hear: Not only marriage, but marital intercourse, was a means of achieving holiness."

When the body of the Church's pronouncements are analyzed, it becomes clear that it was not contraception, per se, that the Church opposed. It was sexual intercourse — *free of the possibility of pregnancy.* Only openness to procreation during each and every sex act could justify sexual relations, could make even marital sex moral. That was the nub of it. The grimmest exponent of that thinking had been St. Augustine in the fifth century, when Christianity resided exclusively in the Catholic Church. His views are said "to have paralyzed Christian thinking in this area for one thousand years." Woman's purpose, he declared, was "to bear children and take care of men when they are old."

But it was not only the ancient popes and saints who described the marital act as "carnal," "lustful," and "shameful." By the middle of the twentieth century, a gigantic chasm had developed between modern Catholic thinking and what was still being taught in the seminary and preached from the pulpit.

Right up to the late 1950s, when the pill was on the market, the most widely used theology book (Noldin) in U.S. Catholic seminaries described the sexual act as "a thing filthy in itself." Another seminary textbook of the same era (Genicot-Salsmans) defined the marriage contract as something which gives people "the right to perform indecent acts." On the parish level, at weeklong instructive sessions, missionary priests threatened Catholic women that if they practiced the shameful sin of "artificial" birth control "the faces of your unborn children will haunt you on your deathbed." When God in the natural scheme of things intended that a child be conceived, then earthly, selfish self-indulgence in sterile sex acts was not to stand in the way. To be a mother was a woman's wifely destiny and her crowning spiritual glory. In heaven, special rewards awaited her if she were true to her conjugal duties. Or, unspeakable punishment, if she were not. Above all, it was to be clearly understood that the primary purpose of the marital sex act was procreation. The ancient pronouncement of Clement of Alexandria was still echoing in the mid-twentieth century. Yet, hairline cracks began to appear in the doctrinal wall. Although Pius XI in his 1931 encyclical *Casti Canubii* flatly condemned all forms of artificial birth control, he did concede it was all right to practice periodic abstinence, even for long periods of time, if for serious reasons a new life should not be created. In 1950 and 1951, his successor, Pius XII, broadened the exceptions to the rule. Though still permitting only "natural" forms of birth control, he approved the rhythm method as a legitimate way to prevent pregnancy. While he emphasized that using rhythm for less than a serious reason was gravely sinful, he recognized medical, eugenic, economic, and social factors as worthy motives. John Rock would turn these "cracks" into gaping holes in the viewpoint of many Church scholars. The old world in which the traditional bans had made sense no longer existed.

On a world scale, ordinary men and women were caught up in great sweeps of change. Life in the industrialized world produced far different pressures in support of birth control than had primitive societies, but there was no respite anywhere. Modern living extended life itself. Fewer babies died. Everyone lived longer. The rising cost of living added inexorably to the cost of rearing children, whose education extended from eight, to twelve to sixteen and twenty years of schooling.

In quality of life the city ghetto began to rival the hopelessness of rural desolation. As populations swelled geometrically, Julian Huxley wrote in 1964, in *The Human Crisis,* that without major checks, the world population would reach four billion by 1980. He underestimated the count. In 1980, the actual world population surpassed 4.5 billion!

The critical problem was that as more millions of human beings survived childhood, there were vastly more people of childbearing age abroad in the world. The worst sting was felt in countries where more and more people were left dependent on less and less arable land. Poverty, famine, illiteracy, mass migration, and internecine warfare could not be far behind, as the tragic course of events has repeatedly proven. Add to that the hideous reality of permanent mental retardation imposed by malnutrition during early childhood and you have a dilemma that has been described as virtually the creation of two species of humans. The present revolution in technology threatens to raise the stakes a whole new order of magnitude between the "haves" and "have-nots" of the next century. Millions more will be shut out of participation in the world of tomorrow.

In the industrialized nations, however, there was remarkable progress. Women were demanding new freedom and status — economically, legally, educationally, and socially. Science revolutionized the understanding of conception, demonstrating the equal role played by the female egg and male sperm. Psychology introduced new insight into the fundamental role played by human sexuality in gender development and personality formation. Sociology and anthropology uncovered broad cultural differences in human sexual and social behavior and backed up these observations with secular, nonjudgmental data. Sexual and marital variations were shown to be neither "right" nor "wrong," but, rather, the reflections of varying tastes, customs, and mores. The human social, sexual relationships proved to be not as cut-and-dried as earlier views would have them.

The birth control debate that boiled over at midcentury was further sharpened by the little recognized factor of the maturation of Catholic universities, which had become centers for bold new social, behavioral, and theological study. The Vatican recognized — within limits — that change was in the wind. In a prophetic statement, Pope Pius XII, in 1946, cautioned that the Church should not be perceived as its authorities — popes, bishops and theologians. He reminded the College of Cardinals that "the laity are the Church." Had Rome been listening to its own voices as well as those of society at large, it would have known by 1957 when the pill was first available (as a menstrual therapy) that new perceptions of human sexuality were emerging that cried out for open-minded consideration. Instead, Rome still seemed largely untouched by the torment of the faithful. The single most all-consuming problem besetting the laity was birth control. For practicing Catholics, the prohibitions were instruments of daily agony: the fear of pregnancy cast against the fear of condemnation to hell.

In that climate there was no getting around the portent of the arrival of the pill. It was the most momentous challenge, as more than one eminent Catholic theologian pointed out, since the most embarrassing previous "scientific" error in Church history: the prosecution of Galileo in 1633 for propounding that the Earth revolved around the sun. Pope Paul VI was cautioned by his own advisers, though he did not heed them, that the Church simply could not afford another "Galileo affair." Before the debate had run its course, the pill in some ways exceeded the Galileo situation. "The Galileo controversy, as important as it was to intellectuals, had nothing to do with what goes on in the beds of married people two or three nights a week, every week of the year," according to Chicago priest-sociologist Father Andrew Greeley, who documented the devastating effect that the Church's final ruling on birth control had on Catholics. The pill not only became a test of the Church's position on birth control, he said, as did others, it led to a rock-bottom reaction that called into question the fundamental authority of the papacy.

Not only was the pill different, so was its foremost proponent, John Rock. He was not a Margaret Sanger to be put down as a scandalous sexmonger, a person who did not know her place, an insult to womanhood and common decency. Nor was he a Paul Blanshard, the prolific, professional-Protestant author, whose credibility in his attacks on Catholicism was largely destroyed by his snide and vitriolic style.

Rock was more than an expert on human reproductive physiology and human sexuality. He was a man steeped in his religion, *his* Roman Catholicism, as well. Beyond and above everything else, he was a man of conscience who was not to be intimidated or denied his convictions. He would stand up for what he thought was right and he was eminently qualified to do so. In an odd sense he'd been getting ready for such a confrontation all his life. His unerring dignity kept the fight on a high plane, making it all the harder for Church figures to put him down. But the challenge to the Church would be different from anything he had ever undertaken. It was not just a question of proving scientific validity. There would be no equivalent of the FDA hearing officer at the Vatican. This time, winning social approval of the pill would require the marshaling of public opinion on a world scale, convincing fellow Catholics to trust their own conscience (as they were bound by their religion to do, though few knew it), and persuading Catholic religious leaders to rethink the meaning and morality of sex according to more enlightened knowledge.

In 1960, when the stage was being set for the confrontation, Rock was a robust, vigorous seventy years old. He had looked death as well as life in the eye many times, personally and with his patients. He was seasoned and confident, canny and wise. And he was that most formidable of persons, an essentially good human being. He wanted first to preserve the family and after that, the family of Man. He knew what he was talking about, medically, maritally, sexually, sociologically, demographically, and theologically. And he was marvelously articulate. He spoke with care as well as candor. And he was enormously likable and believable. The press loved him, recognizing his honesty and reveling in his quotability. He was a force to be reckoned with, the Church soon learned, a remarkably worthy opponent.

From the first salvo, he took on the Church hierarchy on their own turf.

Early in April 1960, a month before the FDA officially approved Enovid as the first oral contraceptive, Rock addressed four hundred obstetricians and gynecologists assembled in Cincinnati at a meeting of the American Society for the Study of Sterility. But sterility was not the main subject on their minds on that occasion. The subject that electrified the meeting was the scientific breakthrough in contraception, the new progestins — the pill. The national medical press corps was present and waiting, well aware that the main issue before the house was not the medical aspects of the pill. The question crackled in the air: What would the Church do now? They knew that, in 1957, Pope Pius XII had sanctioned use of the pill solely for therapeutic reasons — to treat endometriosis or to "regulate" a woman's erratic monthly cycle so she could more reliably practice rhythm. At the sterility society meeting, the national press was lined up to hear how Rock would respond. He didn't disappoint them. With characteristic aplomb, he spoke his mind and took the papal reasoning a critical step forward. As *Time* magazine reported it, "Dr. Rock viewed the pills as merely a means of modifying a woman's monthly cycle. As an active Roman Catholic Dr. Rock went further and provocatively insisted that it must be acceptable to the church as a morally permissible variant of the rhythm method."

A "morally permissible variant of the rhythm method." That was to be the line of reasoning upon which he would base his case for Church acceptance of the pill. It was a masterful strategy, for it was the most vulnerable point in the Church's argument. He repeated the line in dozens of articles, carried in the leading popular magazines of the day — *Saturday Evening Post, Good Housekeeping, Reader's Digest, Redbook,* and in hundreds of newspaper, magazine, radio, and TV interviews. Overnight he became the single most sought-after subject of the public communications media, whose appetite for elaboration of the birth control question seemed insatiable.

Rock not only didn't duck the issue of the Church's opposition, he seemed to enjoy the debate. He also knew enough to take his case to the general public and to state it in terms that concerned them. In one article, published in *Good Housekeeping* in July 1961 and carried in *Reader's Digest* that September, entitled "We Can End the Battle over Birth Control," Rock reached millions of readers in dozens of countries. He wrote, in part:

> As yet, it [the pill] is unique in affording a truly natural method of birth control — the one the body uses to prevent conception — so it should meet no cultural, and eventually overcome present limited religious, objection. This method is obviously much more "natural" than wilful intramarital continence. . . .
>
> Obviously to man's God-given reason, man is not intended to beget young merely to have them die of starvation or violent death after a bare, beastly existence. Reason manifests that man's intellect was provided, among other objectives, to prevent this, but without violating his sexual nature or his marriage (by intramarital continence) through which this is fulfilled. Toward this end, his intellect, I submit, has evolved the pill.
>
> The church hierarchy opposes use of the pill as immoral, but among communicants there is an increasing willingness to accept it. Close to half a million women are using the pill for contraceptive purposes. And it is hard for me to believe these women are all Protestants.

The articles outraged Church leadership, and Rock felt the first sting of what he could expect from that quarter. Typical of their reactions was the retort of the American Jesuit John Lynch in the prestigious journal *Theological Studies.* Lynch cited "misleading lucubrations by John Rock MD" and contended that Rock's statements "illustrate the sort of specious reasoning, unreasoning emotionalism, half-truths and fallacies to which the faithful are being exposed on this elemental question of the oral contraceptive." Lynch said it was a closed issue. He saw "treachery" in any such consideration of the generative function. If the door were opened for one instant, he cautioned, there was no end to the possibilities for abuse of the marital act. In obvious consternation, Lynch recognized that "the pills are now regarded as an effective means of avoiding pregnancy without necessary recourse to even periodic continence." Without intending to do so, Lynch verified that the problem was not, per se, the prevention of conception, but indulgence in sex . . . free of its procreative consequence.

Rock kept a file copy of every commentary by an ecclesiastic on his public statements, just as he did the thousands upon thousands of letters he received from people who wrote after reading his articles. He answered every one, personally. In a July 2, 1962, letter to a Catholic doctor and his brother, who were sympathetic to Rock's point of view, he wrote: "Your brother and you and I apparently think just about the same on this troublesome problem and are convinced that the official Church attitude is the bunk. If you have not seen the latest issue of *Theological Studies* in which Father Lynch of Weston (Mass) roasts me through and through with, what I consider a lot of nonsensical, outworn arguments, you had better not read it. I am sure it would only annoy you. It does, however, make quite clear the job that people as you and your brother and I have ahead of us. Let us keep at it and give it all we've got." What Rock had to give to the job proved to be plenty. He also knew the price he would have to pay.

He knew all too well from past experience what he faced from the entrenched Catholic community. Professional Catholic colleagues in Boston had more than once tried to have him excommunicated. One was Dr. Frederick Good, one-time head of the obstetrical service at Boston City Hospital. While the hospital's medical expertise was unexcelled, the conditions under which its patients were housed and cared for, in Good's era, could be callous and crude. None were worse than those for pregnant women about to deliver, who routinely were hosed down in old soapstone sinks when, as their labor began, their "water broke" and they expelled amniotic fluid. Not until the Civil Rights era of the 1960s did antipoverty activists end such practices. Good and his counterparts were content to use the patients for teaching purposes, providing them usually with expert medical care but ignoring the demeaning conditions under which they received it. Rock considered Good "really one of the stupidest, successful practicing obstetricians in Boston. Yet it was Good who complained very strenuously that I should so boldly receive communion at the Immaculate Conception Church every Sunday . . . ," Rock remembers. The Immaculate Conception not only was the church where Rock and his wife were married, it was an architecturally magnificent church operated by the Jesuit order and considered the intellectual seat of Catholicism in Boston. "I always sat down in one of the side aisles near the altar so I could be by myself and unobtrusively take communion," Rock recalls. "Good spotted me there, so he must have been looking around very thoroughly to even notice me. He thought it was an insult to the Church that such an apostate as I should *flaunt* my Catholicism by receiving communion. He was so stupid, a nitwit really." Good demanded that the then archbishop of Boston, Richard Cardinal Cushing, excommunicate Rock. Good was not the only one. "There was a whole gang of them," Rock said, "but they didn't count for anything with me."

Cushing, a burly giant of a man with an inimitable nasal voice and street accent that bespoke his South Boston Irish background, was not a man easily pushed around, not even by "important" parishioners, like Dr. Good. Often mocked by more learned Catholic scholars, Cushing in his own way was a match for any of them. He was politically suave and essentially good-hearted. In his later years, he healed many of the historic rifts between Protestants, Catholics, and Jews in the city. In Rock's case, Cushing was truly his shepherd and protected him from the Catholic wolves in the archdiocese who wanted to devour him.

"Cushing had no bad feeling toward this man at all. To the contrary, he had a warm spot in his heart for John Rock. He truly liked him and admired him and he was not going to interfere with him in any way," according to Monsignor Francis J. Lally. An urbane and literary man, Lally was editor of the Boston archdiocesan paper, *The Pilot,* during this period, and very much in the style of the new breed of priests. He was also a member of the five-man Boston Redevelopment Authority. Rock and Lally were close friends, often lunching and dining together, and both enjoyed taking part in the Tavern Club's irreverent theatrical productions. "I never saw a man who could move into a room and you would feel as soon as he came in that he was a beloved person. Now that's a rare kind of thing," Lally remembered.

Lally was called to Rock's house immediately after his wife died. "She was upstairs, laid out in her bed. Even then, I remember him speaking to me about his faith. He felt consoled as a Catholic, believing fully that there was an afterlife, that this [world] was not the end. His faith was very strong. I was very impressed by it.

"Later, when people were trying to have him excommunicated, I remember saying to him, 'Aren't you afraid of being thrown out of the Church?' He said, 'Not the least bit afraid. Never. There's no way they can throw me out. The Church belongs to me as much as to anyone, including the pope. I was baptized in it and I'm going to die in it. They can't throw me out. I'll be a Catholic all my life and I'll be a Catholic in eternal life.' I thought there again, he showed himself to be a man of complete faith. He knew what he believed and he was not going to be deterred by any ecclesiastical folderol. They were not going to be able to excommunicate him or suspend him or give him penalties or do anything else to him. He just wouldn't accept them. He said, 'They have no power over me. I belong in the Church. No one can put me out of it.' " Lally also was Cushing's spokesman. As such, he was very close to the cardinal and was in a position to know that conservatives at St. John's Seminary (on the grounds of the cardinal's residence) also were after Rock's hide. But Cushing ignored them. He was not insensitive to what Rock was trying to accomplish, nor was he unaware that if Rock succeeded in changing the Church's position on birth control, some of the credit would accrue to Cushing himself. He let Rock be.

Caring for his wife during her ordeal with cancer took precedence over everything in his life for a while, including Rock's jousting with the Church over the pill. But after her death on August 9, 1961, and after he had rallied from the first terrible despair of her loss, he decided what he must and would do. He would write a book, presenting his case in no uncertain terms for Roman Catholic acceptance of the pill. He would write, as he always did, with passion as well as compassion, scholarship, close reasoning, and his unrivaled capacity for plain talk.

The foundation for Rock's thesis (and in time that of some Catholic theologians) that the Church might accept the pill was a succession of statements by Pope Pius XII. In October 1951, Pius XII in an address to Catholic midwives had recognized that there might be serious motives — medical, eugenic, economic, and social — for avoiding procreation. If such "indications" existed, the pope said, "it follows that observance of the sterile period can be licit." He approved rhythm!

A month later he expanded upon the point while addressing two Italian societies, the Association of Large Families and the Family Front society. He declared: "We have affirmed the lawfulness and at the same time the limits — in truth quite broad — of a regulation of offspring. . . . Science, it may be hoped, will develop for this method a sufficiently secure base." It was significant that the pope used the term "regulation." It was a long step forward from earlier papal condemnations of any means of contraception. And in 1958, Pius XII, addressing the Seventh International Congress of Hematology, officially sanctioned use of the pill "not to prevent conception but only on the advice of a doctor as a necessary remedy because of a disease of the uterus or organism." In other words, to treat endometriosis, excessive and painful menstrual bleeding. Part of the implicit reason for this was to allow pill usage to regulate erratic menstrual cycles. This would, it was theorized, strengthen the reliability of the sanctioned rhythm method of birth control.

These papal proclamations were to provide the wedge, philosophically, that Rock hoped to use to drive home his message. If sexual relations were moral during a woman's nonfertile time during the menstrual cycle, then why should they be immoral because the pill, by mimicking nature, prolonged that time? It was illogical, if not ridiculous, to his thinking, to reason otherwise. The job to be done was to get the message across on a grand scale. To get people thinking about it on familiar terms. To lead them to do so. A book, he felt, the *right* book, could do it.

He put himself on the line with every sentence, beginning with the title *The Time Has Come: A Catholic Doctor's Proposals to End the Battle Over Birth Control*. It was published in the spring of 1963 by Alfred A. Knopf, a New York publishing house. In a single shot, like David's biblical rock against Goliath, the book's message reverberated around the world. It was translated into French, German, and Dutch, and sold abroad even more briskly than in the United States, both in hard cover and paperback. It was perceived as exactly what it was, a head-on challenge to the Holy See in Rome.

Rock's old Harvard classmate Christian Herter, twice governor of Massachusetts and national secretary of state, wrote the foreword for Rock's outspoken work. It touched Rock deeply that Herter, nearly fifty years after their Harvard days, would publicly champion his cause. Herter, a Republican and the living embodiment of Yankee, Brahmin Boston, had returned to Washington in the early 1960s to serve as presidential adviser on foreign trade to the nation's first Catholic president, another Bostonian and Harvard alumnus, John F. Kennedy. In the foreword to Rock's book, Herter wrote in part:

> Perhaps someone other than John Rock could have written this book, but I doubt it. Fate seems inexorably to assign certain critical tasks to certain individuals. . . . John Rock does not appear on the roster of fame; his distinction is known mainly to his colleagues in medicine and science and to his intimate friends. Yet evidently he was destined to be a point of intersection for certain great forces and principles which have impaled him on the horns of a very personal dilemma: A Roman Catholic immensely devoted to his church, a physician more than nominally loyal to the Hippocratic Oath, he is a gynecologist whose concern for the health of his patients and their families led him to become a key participant in the development of the world's first efficient oral contraceptive. Another factor in his background, which has impelled him further, is one that I share: As citizens of Massachusetts we have both been concerned with the wasteful and protracted struggle over birth control in that state. . . .
>
> He has chosen not to escape from the painful horn of conflict between Catholics and non-Catholics over birth control, but to grasp it and to search doggedly for ways to resolve this chronic dispute.
>
> This would be an important book if it dealt, as it does so well, just with the half century of strife over birth control in the United States. But he recognizes how the population crisis makes it not just desirable but urgently necessary to terminate the birth control acrimony globally as well as nationally.

With his customary eloquent simplicity, Rock explained in the preface why he felt he must speak out:

> With increasing frequency, I was disturbed by the realization that the voice of my conscience was not always telling me what the priests of my Church kept saying were its dictates regarding human reproductive function — what was right and what was wrong in how a person willed, or permitted or prevented expression of his God-given sexuality. Only stupidity or callous blindness through decades of dealing with marital situations and of facilitating the creation and delivery of new life . . . could prevent the formulation of realistic thoughts on the nature of human sexuality. . . .
>
> It is easy to think in the abstract of omnipotence, omniscience, omnipresence, even of all-pervasive trust. It is easy to imagine the utter

necessity — yes, the inevitability of complete submission to the Creator to whom these qualities pertain. I suggest it is not easy for any descendant of Adam to achieve this complete submission.

Not feeling his God-given sexuality, not feeling the urge to escape as many of the handicaps as possible by withdrawing from the world — from all worldliness, from all society — as have many of every known religion, I must perforce face up to them.

He first argued for understanding of love and sexual behavior, speaking always from his years of long intimacy professionally (and personally) with the subject.

Every language throughout the world has a collective name for it; ours is "love." . . . Love is now recognized to be part of the human sex instinct, equal to the coital impulse in psychological significance . . . human sexual relations without love become inadequate for full satisfaction and love without coitus at mutually agreeable intervals becomes frustrating and ultimately demoralizing. Love fused by coitus, but without children to bring up, lacks completion; but when it brings more children than can properly be cared for, it is dangerously strained, even distorted. . . . Such is what, after forty years as a Catholic obstetrician-gynecologist, student and teacher, I have found to be the nature of human sexuality.

He argued how near together, rather than separated, the various Christian churches were on birth control; and he stressed the new thinking of Catholic, as well as non-Catholic, authorities on the meaning of marriage. He cited Catholic dissertations on "natural law that contended modern interpretations of St. Thomas Aquinas' writings on natural law would be unrecognizable to Aquinas." Above all, Rock cited Aquinas' view that it is "natural" for man to use his reason to solve problems with which a blind and irrational nature confronts him.

He spelled out the natural hormonal governance over the timing of fertility in women and how the pill prevented reproduction "by modifying the time sequences in the body's own functions. It has been my consistent feeling that when properly used for conception control, they merely serve as adjuncts to nature," he wrote, conceding that many Catholic moralists "certainly do not share my belief."

"My reasoning," he went on, "is based in part on the fact that the rhythm method, which is sanctioned by the Church, depends precisely on the secretion of progesterones from the ovaries, which action these compounds merely duplicate. It is progesterone, in the healthy woman, that prevents ovulation and establishes the pre- and post-menstrual 'safe period.' The physiology underlying the spontaneous 'safe period' is identical to that initiated by the steroid compounds and is equally harmless to the individual. Indeed, the use of the compounds for fertility control may be characterized as a 'pill-established safe period' and would seem to carry the same implications."

He combated the idea, expounded by some Catholic doctors and clergy, that the pills were sterilizing agents. To the contrary, they tended to increase fertility when a woman ceased using them. He noted that three Vatican theologians had concluded that it was all right for women, specifically nuns in the Congo, in danger of rape to use the pill. This sanctioned use was based on the point that victims of rape do not have the alternative of sexual abstention to which married couples can resort to avoid conception. Rock's counterquestion — "Could a wife in imminent danger of a rapacious attack by a husband follow the same rule that applies to her maiden sister?" — was considered radical at the time. It hardly would be so today, in light of criminal rape charges filed by wives against husbands.

But unquestionably, the point on which Rock scored most directly was that surrounding sex and love. The Church made many statements, he stressed, that "condemn the use of the pill . . . for the subjective intent to avoid conception . . . that sex may be used, perhaps only for love. Does such an attitude easily conform with the Church's justification of the rhythm method?" he asked, tellingly. "The Papal documents sanctioning rhythm refer explicitly to the licitness of satisfying (by coitus) the secondary ends of marriage — sexual harmony and the allaying of concupiscence — when procreation should be avoided for serious reasons. Is this not a regard for sexual expression as a completely independent good, totally apart from procreation?" Should means be discovered, as some Church leaders, including the pope, had begun to urge, for the simple, accurate prediction of ovulation "to make rhythm more reliable," did not that imply that it would be used to produce "exactly the same interference as do the oral pills, separating sexual expression as an independent good from procreation?" Rock insisted upon knowing. "I am persuaded that the Church has not concluded its examination of the morality of the progestational steroids when used for fertility control."

Rock pulled out all the stops in the book. He led the reader through terrifying statistics on population growth and then pulled them back to actual cases where fear of Catholic repercussions (most of them well founded) had outrageously interfered with providing birth control protection (usually the fitting of a diaphragm) for even non-Catholic women in big city hospitals. His examples showed how extensively this happened, even in states which had no anti–birth control laws. The most flagrant was the 1958 attempt in New York City where Dr. Louis Hellman, the director of obstetrics at Kings County Hospital, a municipal hospital with a huge obstetric service, was stopped from fitting a diaphragm for a diabetic woman. She was a Protestant with three children, whose two previous pregnancies were delivered by cesarean section — a woman, Rock wrote, "whose life would unquestionably be endangered by another pregnancy." After two months of front-page news reports in New York's papers, including *New York Times* editorial support, Rock wrote, "a more comprehensive picture of the current political and religious status of contraception than had ever been seen before" emerged. An investigation showed that the stop order issued by the commissioner of hospitals for New York City had been instigated by the chancery office of the archdiocese of New York. The issue was finally resolved with the adoption of a resolution that permitted New York's municipal hospitals to provide birth control help for women "whose life and health" may be jeopardized by pregnancy. The wording of the permit is far more limited, of course, than today's authorizations for abortion, but it was a breakthrough for the times.

Rock cast all his comments on such cases in apologetic terms, noting that attitudes were changing within, as well as outside, the Catholic Church. He contended that such conflicts grew out of stereotyped ideas of the Church's true position. He wrote: "As Monsignor J. D. Conway said of Catholic opposition to the New York hospital settlement, 'such a course is but the rear-guard action of a battle which has been lost all over the country.' " Rock called for new research to make rhythm more reliable by finding a way reliably to predict or induce ovulation. He urged major new government programs be created to bring birth control aid to developing countries. And he pleaded passionately for a new era of reconciliation between the Catholic Church and all others over birth control "to work for a solution for all."

Had the Church Fathers been listening, truly listening, they might have seen that in Rock they had the champion they needed. He preached family love, monogamy, fidelity, responsibility, the nurturing of spousal bonds, duty to the rearing and education of children.

His book hit the market like an explosive. Rather than merely being reviewed, its arrival made headlines in news stories and was the topic of leading columnists in newspapers and magazines across the country and the world. While the book passed from hand to hand to a remarkable extent, sales were not dramatic.

As Margaret Sanger well knew, "a cause is won by its enemies." The reaction of the Catholic Church to Rock's book could not have been more helpful to Rock's challenge.

In Cleveland, Monsignor Francis W. Carney, director of the Family Life Bureau of the Cleveland Catholic diocese called Rock "a moral rapist, using his strength as a man of science to assault the faith of his fellow Catholics." He also attacked Rock's suggestion that Catholics should follow their own conscience on the question of birth control. Rather than writing misleading books, Carney said, "one would hope and pray that Dr. Rock would concentrate his research on a method to detect ovulation and thus spare his church the necessity of correcting his views." Monsignor Carney concluded that Catholics were taking "a bum rap" for the population explosion. Monsignor George A. Kelly, director of the Family Life Bureau of the Archdiocese of New York and author of the *Catholic Marriage Manual,* thundered: "A thousand years from now we may be eating meat on Friday, but at that time murder, adultery and contraception will still be sins. These latter involve God's law and not even the Pope nor even a large number of sinning couples can turn wrong into right. The reason why artificial prevention of births is immoral is written into the very nature of the sexual organs and the marital act itself. The sex organs were made by God to reproduce the human race." Kelly called Rock "a man who capitalizes on his Catholicism, yet speaks not at all out of a Catholic conscience. He knows that contraception is, for the Catholic, an intrinsically evil thing, yet he writes as if it is merely a passing Catholic fad." Kelly decried attempts by advocates of contraception "to make government at all levels, a sub-department of the Planned Parenthood Federation of America."

Catholic doctors were enlisted to write of the dangers of the pill to women's health, to family stability, and to morality. They raised wild prospects of women postponing menopause via pill use and then being fertile and pregnant in their sixties. They warned of the psychological damage in the pill to husbands who no longer could impregnate their wives at will. And while couching their warnings in terms of protecting women, they simultaneously belittled them by doubting whether women were up to the task of remembering to take a pill daily. Although public funds could not be used for family planning, one Catholic physician used his position as state commissioner of public health to publish and disseminate a booklet citing moral as well as physical dangers in the pill.

Over and over, prominent American Catholic clergymen quoted back at Rock what he already well knew — the papal line that the pill was not "licit" for overt contraceptive use. But each time the Catholic press castigated Rock, the stories of course were publicizing his book and his position. And scores more people looked into it.

Rarely has the news media made so much of a new book. Of course, it wasn't the book itself that attracted the attention. Rather it was the open challenge posed by a prominent Catholic personage and an unsurpassed expert in his field. *Life, Time,* and *Newsweek* all carried major stories. United Press International religion writer Louis Cassels said, "The book ought to be read by every church leader, politician and plain citizen who is concerned about the problem of limiting population growth." His syndicated column appeared in papers across the country. The *New York Herald Tribune* called the book "a work that may turn out to be a truly historic document."

Life magazine carried a five-page spread entitled "A Catholic Doctor Speaks Up," including full-page photos of Rock with his (then) seventeen grandchildren gathered for Easter festivities at the family home in Brookline. Other photos showed Rock leaving daily mass at St. Mary's Church, in Brookline. In that article, too, Rock pulled no punches. On religion, in the *Life* interview, Rock said, "Changing Catholic Church positions from the outside is like David fighting Goliath, except David won. I am not David. I seek to change the Church's position from inside." Of the world population problem he said, "When anything really threatens humanity, the Church steps up to face it."

That August, the *New York Times* featured on its front page a four-part series called "Catholics and Birth Control" by its religion editor, George Barrett. The extraordinary series, heralding for the first time what had unofficially become known as the birth control "debate," illustrates the prominence that Rock — and a handful of new "liberal" Catholic spokesmen — had won for the subject. Barrett painstakingly showed how divided Catholics — both lay and clergical — were on the practice of birth control. He documented the still small but significant acceptance of birth control by Catholics in the United

States and Europe. He cast this against the bitter campaigns against birth control still being waged in less developed but heavily Catholic countries, like Puerto Rico, "one of the most densely packed areas on this globe."

Of Rock's role, Barrett wrote, "The excitement in Catholic circles over Dr. Rock's book and in fact Dr. Rock's decision to write it, reflect the ferment that has been stirring the Catholic Church on the subject of birth control." Barrett noted that more than a hundred years ago, John Henry Newman, an Oxford scholar, philosopher, theologian, and later Cardinal of the Roman Catholic Church, was accused of fallacy. "For many years John Newman lived sub luce maligna — under a dark light, as the theologians interpret the Latin — before he was vindicated," Barrett pointed out. He added, "A few weeks ago an eminent priest-theologian of the Catholic church directed some words of his own to another 'heretic' — Dr. John Rock. 'Tell John,' said the priest-theologian softly, 'that there are things I can't put into my writing, but please remind him of Cardinal Newman. Tell him, please, that when things get rough to take courage, to remember the Newmans of the Catholic Church; tell him to remember that there have been others before him in our church who have also had to live sub luce maligna — for a while.'"

As if those public displays were not enough to thoroughly rankle Catholic officials, Rock next became the darling of network television. In May of 1962, before the book was published, he had appeared on a special *CBS Reports* telecast, "Birth Control and the Law." When the book came out, in an unprecedented TV action at the time, CBS updated the program to include references to his book and reran the show in May 1963. Not to be outdone, NBC developed an hour-long documentary, hosted by David Brinkley, which was shown in November 1963. The Brinkley show virtually took a viewer for a walk through Rock's book. It opened with Rock and Brinkley riding around Rock's home town of Marlborough, in a horse-drawn carriage, while Rock recalled the advice given him as a teenager by the local priest about "keeping his own conscience." The program moved along to show Rock in his medical practice at the Rock Reproductive Clinic, counseling women who were desperate to have children and those who had too many. At its conclusion, Rock was seen, seated at his desk, answering personally each and every letter written to him by the thousands of people who had read the book, news stories, or had seen him on TV. With typical aplomb, he read a few that were far from complimentary. He read aloud one from an angry Catholic woman who excoriated him for his stand, saying "you should be afraid to meet your Maker." Rock wrote back, cordially but pointedly, "My dear Madam, in my faith, we are taught that the Lord is with us always. When my time comes, there will be no need for introductions."

The Church was right about Rock in one regard. He indeed was a force to be reckoned with. In the TV shows, especially, shows viewed by tens of millions of Americans, Rock came across at his best: informed, concerned, kindly, committed, honest, forthright, and yet full of humor and understanding. He was a television talkmaster's dream interview. He knew his subject, but he wasn't pedantic. He spoke with wisdom and warmth at the same time. He exuded confidence and he called forth from the viewer absolute trust. His stage and lecture experience stood him in marvelous stead; he knew how to carry off a good line, and he did it with longstanding grace. His message carried as none other from the laity ever had.

A front-row observer of the developments of the day was the Redemptorist Father Francis X. Murphy who had reported the background and happenings of Vatican II for *The New Yorker* under the nom de plume Xavier Rynne. A strong and early advocate for change in the Church's unyielding position on birth control, Murphy said that Rock's book found the chink in the wall of the Church's opposition. "It was Rock's book, more than any other single factor, that confronted Rome. Rock contended that the use of the anovulants was equivalent to a 'pill-established safe period' and would seem to carry the same moral specifications. It was a thought-provoking analogy. Most theologians rejected Rock's position — at least publicly. But in keeping with Rock's contention, he began to reach significant voices within the fold. Quite soon, some European theologians and bishops defended the pill to regulate birth." Their statements were a far cry from the temperate response of Cardinal Cushing in Boston, who said "there is much that is good in this book" but beyond that declared Rock off base in his thinking that the pill could be accepted.

Murphy was far from alone in his conviction that it was Rock — and his book — that turned the tide for consideration of the pill as an acceptable contraceptive by Rome.

In his authoritative work on the history of contraception in the Catholic Church, John Noonan points out:

In the seven years from the beginning of the debate on anovulants (from 1956 when they were first reported) no theologians had defended their lawfulness to regulate fertility except in special cases of correction of the cycle and in lactation. (For four years since 1958 when Pius XII permitted their use for therapeutic purposes only, his statement had been taken as all-controlling.)

In 1963 this situation was drastically altered. The change began with a book entitled *The Time Has Come* . . . Rock's thesis was immediately rejected by several American theologians — Connell, Lynch, Ford, and Kelly — who commented on it. In the Netherlands, [however,] individuals had, since 1960, doubted the teaching on the pill. In 1963 in a television speech, William Bekkers, bishop of 's-Hertogenbosch, noted that it was unclear whether the traditional statements applied to the progesterone pill. These pills were not contraceptives in the usual sense.

More uncertainty followed in the Netherlands until August 1963 (five months after Rock's book was published), when the seven bishops of the Netherlands, acting as a national hierarchy, officially declared that "new views of man and his existence of sexuality and conjugal love, as well as new means for fertility control confront the Church with new questions." Even if the pill should not be a "generally used" solution, the bishops held that "in special situations, the use of these means might be accepted." They hoped the question would be discussed more at the next session of the Vatican Council. The Dutch thus left open the question of the "licitness" of the pill as an acceptable contraception.

Next to pick up Rock's challenge was Louis Janssens, a theologian at the University of Louvain. Janssens had earlier argued that the pill was different, and never condemned its use. Now, he raised a new question that Murphy considered "ominous" for the continued ban on the pill. Time is an important factor in human acts, Janssens pointed out. When one changed the time that one performed an act, one introduced human calculation into it. If preventing conception by the timing of sexual relations during sterile periods under the rhythm method was legitimate, why isn't the pill legitimate? Janssens asked. It merely extended the woman's nonfertile time. Almost simultaneously two other theologians, both Dutch Dominicans, also concluded it was lawful for Catholics to use the pill to regulate births.

Suddenly, Noonan reported, "the pill became the center and symbol of effort to modify the Catholic position on birth control." Rock's book had given impetus to an open challenge. To cap it off, in April 1964 the former archbishop of Bombay, Thomas D. Roberts, in a major article published in the London *Times,* openly questioned the rationality of the entire Catholic position on contraception in general. Roberts's position set off an explosive reaction in England, prompting the archbishop of Westminster, John Heenan, to declare publicly in the name of all the bishops of England and Wales that "Contraception ... is not an open question, for it is against the law of God." The seven bishops of the Netherlands and the twenty-three of England and Wales were now in open contradiction!

Reaction was not limited to Catholics by any means. Instead, non-Catholics found for the first time that doors were open for discussion — and better yet, action — to a degree that would have been impossible only a few years earlier. It was more than heartening, it was thrilling for them to find prominent Catholics and Catholic institutions receptive to the idea that together they might establish a new common ground for birth control.

Many of the meetings were unpublicized, but in the late spring of 1963, only weeks after Rock's book was published, an exploratory meeting was held in the Renaissance chambers of the Vatican between Catholic Church dignitaries and Donald B. Straus, chairman of the Planned Parenthood Federation. Another series of meetings was held, under the spectacular leadership of Father Theodore Hesburgh, president of the University of Notre Dame, on the campus in South Bend, Illinois. The off-the-record sessions brought together theologians, demographers, political scientists, medical researchers, and included some of the Catholic theologians from the great liberal movements in Belgium, France, the Netherlands, West Germany, and parts of Canada. In yet another closed meeting — this one at the Ford Foundation — that bespoke a new tone of good will, steroid chemists, reproduction endocrinologists, and other experts — Catholic and non-Catholic — explored the possibility of a more effective rhythm method.

For Rock, one of the most treasured triumphs came at the hands of John F. Kennedy, America's first Catholic president. Rock had been cruelly disappointed that Kennedy's predecessor, President Dwight D. Eisenhower, a Protestant, had ruled out birth control dissemination as a governmental responsibility, saying, "That's not our business." Kennedy, however, in the early summer of 1963, announced his support for any effort by the government to provide information on population control to "nations requesting it." He also said that the United States "certainly could support" increased research in fertility and human reproduction as well as programs to make the results more available to the world, so that everyone can make their own judgment." Three weeks later, the United States announced a grant of $500,000 to the World Health Organization for those purposes — the first such grant in American history.

Only three men have known the role John Rock played in changing the UN's attitude on birth control. Dr. John Snyder, former dean of the Harvard School of Public Health, is one of them. "In 1962, the World Health Organization met in Geneva. Though we were supposed to be addressing other subjects, the air was full of talk about population, which had been an almost taboo subject. The director of the WHO at the time was Dr. Marcelino Candau, a Brazilian Catholic, who was a suave, skillful, thoughtful politician. He very much wanted to get the subject of family planning on the agenda, but was understandably nervous about doing so because Brazil is a Catholic country. I thought maybe John Rock could be the person to persuade the World Health Organization, through Candau, to get involved. Early the next year, I heard Candau was coming to the United States to get an honorary degree. I was able to intercept him to come to a dinner of the Society of Fellows at the Harvard faculty club in Cambridge. John Rock's book in galley proofs had just arrived on the scene. I cajoled Rock into letting me stuff a set of the galleys in Candau's briefcase. I also managed to get them off to one side to talk together privately, as professionals concerned with the population threat and as one Catholic to another. Candau left with Rock's galleys in his hands, eager to read them. Within six months, Candau appointed a World Health Organization committee on human reproduction, which was the force that led to their change of policy. It was a very significant move. Once Candau had spent that time with Rock and had Rock's book to support him, he no longer felt as isolated as he had previously, as one prominent Catholic advocating something his Church was against. He took great courage from Rock and his book."

In another unexpected and highly unorthodox move for the time, Georgetown University in Washington, D.C., created a center for population and birth control research. It was the brainchild of a Catholic economist, Dr. Donald J. O'Connor, who had been driven to action by his observations of the squalid conditions and human tragedies wrought by overpopulation in Puerto Rico where he served as an economic adviser to the government. O'Connor recruited Dr. Benedict J.

Duffy, a restless and dynamic member of the medical faculty at George-town, to support the project. Duffy, who later became one of Rock's most ardent and steadfast friends, helped to usher the center into existence, initially funded by a grant from the Ford Foundation and an endowment from the Joseph P. and Rose Fitzgerald Kennedy Foundation. He became its first director. Ironically his first major research project for the center irrefutably proved the wide swings and erratic fluctuations of the female menstrual cycle, thereby undermining any hope for an easy approach to improving the rhythm method of birth control.

The Church found no surcease from the subject, even in the Catholic publications. Wilfred Sheed, an associate editor of *Jubilee,* a middle-of-the-road Catholic magazine, wrote of Rock in the summer of 1963: "It would be easy to tick off [Dr. Rock's] foibles and run rings around his amateur theology. It would be easy to dismiss his book. But if it is true, as I think it is, that he voices the grief and irritation of thousands, to dismiss his book is to dismiss them."

Nor was there real escape within the Church itself. Leo Josef Cardinal Suenens, primate of Belgium, and leader of the "progressives" in Rome's Sacred College of Cardinals, bluntly and publicly asked "whether many people . . . do not fall away from the Church because of birth control?" Catholic surveys of Western industrialized countries reported the same birth rates for Catholic as non-Catholic societies. Citing France as an example, Cardinal Suenens went on to observe that "contraception has made a telling incursion into the country's way of life." The Reverend Thomas J. Casey, writing in the *American Catholic Sociological Review,* saw no reason to doubt one study that showed, "for Catholic couples who were married for at least 10 years and still fecund, one out of two practiced a method of birth control forbidden by the church."

Birth control was rapidly becoming the most serious problem the Church had to contend with. Many Catholics were staying away from church. More and more often parish priests reported that in greater number they had to deny otherwise faithful Catholics the sacraments because they insisted upon using artificial methods of contraception. While most continued to go to church, they did not go in peace, one report said: they went in guilt.

The Right Reverend Monsignor George W. Casey, pastor of St. Brigid's church in Lexington, Massachusetts, and a homespun author of a column for the *Boston Herald Traveler,* summed it up. The eighth among ten children himself, Casey recalled that much "of the fire went out" of his sermons on birth control when "I handled the case of a poor, hapless sort of mother who bore her fifth set of twins in as many years and her husband 'took it on the lam.' We are not calling for radical change but room for maneuvering. Families can't raise children the way our parents did."

The hue and cry finally reached the Holy See. Rome simply could not remain silent. The historic moment came on June 23, 1964. As *Newsweek* described it, "the setting was informal. Twenty-seven cardinals had come to Pope Paul VI's private library on the second floor of the Vatican Palace to greet the Pontiff on the eve of the Feast of St. John the Baptist, the saint after whom he had been christened 66 years earlier as Giovanni Battista."

He disclosed to them — and to the world — that he had created a special commission, its membership a secret, to study the birth control question. Called the Papal Commission on Population, the Family and Natality, it marked the first time in Church history that a special study commission had been created to examine an issue in response to world clamor. He said:

> The problem, everyone talks of it, is that of birth control, as it is called, namely of population increases on one hand, and family morality on the other.
> It is an extremely grave problem. It touches on the mainsprings of human life. . . . The question is being subjected to study, as wide and profound as possible, as grave and honest as it must be on a subject of such importance. . . . We will therefore soon give the conclusions of it in the form which will be considered most adapted to the subject and to the aim to be achieved. . . .

Until a decision was reached, Pope Paul said, the general ban on birth control remained in effect, with the exception of rhythm and the pill for therapeutic purposes.

Rock had done it and everyone knew it. He had inspired hundreds of thousands of rank-and-file Catholics to knock on the door of Rome, an unprecedented action. He had given them confidence in their ability — and their right — to decide for themselves whether or not to have a child and when to do it. And he had given them the means to manage it. "The specific issue moving the church away from traditional opposition to all forms of artificial birth control," proclaimed *Newsweek* magazine, "is the new oral contraceptive pills."

If the play given the papal announcement by the news media is used as a yardstick to measure the event, the outcome is graphically obvious. *Newsweek* magazine ran John Rock's picture on the cover, and touted the story as "Birth Control, The Pill and the Church." A photograph of Pope Paul, seated on the papal throne, was carried deep inside. "The meaning of the Pope's statement is clear," *Newsweek* said, noting:

> Not since the Copernicans suggested in the sixteenth century that the sun was the center of the planetary system has the Roman Catholic church found itself on such a perilous collision course with a new body of knowledge. . . . The spectacle of the church leadership following its flock and responding to pressures from below cannot soon be forgotten. . . .

10

THE CHURCH SAYS "NO"

IT was indeed a vain hope on Pope Paul's part that he, or anyone, could stop discussion of the pill or, as an extension, of the birth control question, while the special papal commission deliberated. Looking back, it is nearly impossible to recreate the intensity of world interest in both matters. Only the issue of abortion today evokes comparable controversy and fervor. The Holy See had to contend with seeing much of the ferment emanating from its own doorstep — from the closely reported workings of the papal commission and of the Ecumenical Council, Vatican II. Farther from home, John Rock was not letting up, either. Though nearly seventy-five years old, he was indefatigable, criss-crossing the United States and the Western world to give lectures for both scientists and laymen. In scores of talks and published articles, he kept the spotlight of public attention on the subject. Meanwhile, the pill itself, as it moved into daily usage on a scale unprecedented for any medication, became the object of large research studies. Considering the millions of users, some of the growing concern for the safety of the pill was clearly warranted, but some was exaggerated, it seemed, more as a result of moral indignation than medical probity.

"We now come to October 29, [1964,] a date to be remembered," reported the then Oblate Gregory Baum of Toronto, who was a theological adviser to the Ecumenical Council.

Three Cardinals — Ruffini, Leger and Suenens and the 87-year-old Greek Patriarch, Maximos, insisted that the Church must re-examine its theology of marriage and human sexuality. During these speeches, the Council was spell-bound, electrified. Cardinal [Leo Josephs] Suenens spoke with passion. He pleaded with the bishops not to be afraid of re-examining the traditional position. We do not want another Galileo case, he shouted, one is enough for the Church. Patriarch Maximos [Saigh] insisted that today the Church teaches one thing and the majority of the faithful do another.

The speeches were received with great applause, contrary to regulation. The impression of these speeches in Rome on the same day cannot be exaggerated. The reaction . . . went through the world press; this is a turning point, this is a watershed — we are free to examine the meaning of sexuality in married life according to God's plan of salvation.

Suenens and Maximos had even more to say. Suenens told his brother bishops, "The problem confronts us not because the faithful try to satisfy their passions and egotism, but because thousands of them try with anguish to live in double fidelity, to the doctrine of the Church and to the demands of conjugal and parental love." Maximos was equally blunt. Birth control, he said, "is an urgent problem because it lies at the root of a great crisis in Catholic conscience. There is a question here of a break between the official doctrine of the Church and the contrary practices of the immense majority of Christian couples. Are we not entitled to ask if certain positions [of the Church] are not the outcome of outmoded ideas, and perhaps, a bachelor psychosis on the part of those unacquainted with this sector of life?"

The bishops were not altogether taken by surprise at the unusually forceful pleas that the Church reexamine her position on birth control. Each member of Vatican II had received a copy of a letter signed by more than one hundred lay people, all well-known men of science (including Rock), publishers, teachers, and lawyers. Nor were the bishops of one mind about the propriety of some of their colleagues making such direct and overt calls for change. Archbishop Heenan of England struck out, publicly, at "the few theologians who make a lot of noise in the world and confuse the faithful."

Pope Paul's Papal Commission on Population, the Family and Natality, which everywhere became known as the Birth Control Commission, was a formal outgrowth of the one originated far more quietly by Pope John XXIII a month before his death. The full commission's very existence raised hope by Catholics and non-Catholics alike that great change was imminent. On their own, without waiting for the final decision from Rome, Catholics began to practice birth control in astonishing numbers. Father Andrew Greeley, in a major study for the Catholic-funded National Opinion Research Center in Chicago, found that between 1960 and 1965 (the end of the Ecumenical Council) the use of unapproved forms of birth control increased from 38 to 51 percent among American Catholics (men and women), with almost all of the change accounted for by the invention of the pill. When Catholic women alone were polled, he found in 1965 that 77 percent of those under forty-five were practicing some form of contraception with only 28 percent still relying on the Church-approved rhythm method.

"The development of the pill created a new moral situation which the church would have had to deal with whether or not there had been a Vatican Council," he concluded. "All of the increased nonconformity involved the use of the pill and much of it resulted from the replacement of rhythm by the pill. It would appear that a large number of Catholic women made up their minds that the pill was more effective and no less moral. Indeed, the women who were using the pill" his poll showed, "were *more* likely to receive communion at least once a month than those who practiced rhythm or no method."

Although the commission's membership was never officially revealed by the Vatican, news media followed every development. Catholic news publications made it a full-time occupation. Shortly after Pope Paul enlarged the commission, which was chaired by Archbishop Leo Binz of St. Paul, Minnesota, the *National Catholic Reporter,* a well-regarded and widely read news weekly, published the names of the commission's fifty-seven members. They included theologians, bishops, and lay people (among them married couples) who were recognized experts in theology, medicine, psychology, and demography. They came from all continents and twenty nations. To the pope's credit, he sought a mix of advisers including those known to question the Church's position. Rock, however, was noticeably excluded.

The commission held its first meeting in Rome in March 1965, housed secretly at the Collegio San Jose. From the beginning, the mood of the commission favored the pill. It was known that only seven members wanted to hold the line, adhering to the traditional rhythm-only position. Six members were known to favor outright contraception by any means. The remaining forty-four sought to find in the pill a middle-ground solution.

In reaction to a secret 83-page draft of a preliminary report, outlining three disparate points of view but strongly supporting a change in the birth control prohibitions, Pope Paul added more theologians of a traditional bent to the commission. Then, accused of trying to tip the scales, he added an equal number of revisionists. Still troubled, in February 1966, he again reorganized the commission by naming fifteen cardinals and bishops to act as an executive committee. With this maneuver, he also made the previous commission members consultants to the new hierarchal executive committee.

By the end of June 1966, the commission (including the executive committee) submitted its final reports to the Pope. They were kept absolutely confidential; no hint of their content was disclosed officially. The suspense, worldwide, was enormous. In a last ditch, all-out lobbying effort, the American editor and publisher Cass Canfield, who at the time was president of the Planned Parenthood Federation of America, circulated a carefully researched white paper on birth control as it related to the Church's historic positions. Canfield also made a multistop tour of Europe to confer with lay and religious leaders who were known to carry weight with the commission members and the Vatican.

In October of 1966 there was a wild flurry of excitement as the commission's executive secretary, Father de Riedmatten, predicted that the Vatican would change "its two-thousand-year-old ban on contraception." Speculation grew that Pope Paul would use the occasion, later that month, of the Italian Association of Obstetricians and Gynecologists special audience to make the announcement. Instead the Pope begged for more time, but he gave the first small hint his decision might not be favorable. Soon afterwards a "planted" editorial in *La Osservatore Romano,* the Vatican's paraofficial newspaper, also boded unfavorably. The editorial suggested that the moral solution to the population problem was "mastery of self." The waiting for a decision dragged on.

The world of Rock and the pill did not, of course, stand still while Rome pondered the matter. During the mid-1960s Rock drove himself at a ferocious pace. He averaged thirty personal appearances a year, granted innumerable interviews, and prepared a dozen or more major articles. He wrote and rewrote each one, giving each its own emphasis, but the same theme threaded through them all. In a reflective essay, "Sex, Science and Survival," prepared as the seventh Oliver Bird Lecture and presented at the London School of Hygiene and Tropical Medicine in 1963, he summed up his lifetime conclusions on the true nature of human sexuality. He intended it to be the basis of a sequel to his book, *The Time Has Come,* because, he says, "too many sacerdotes still confused the incredibly profound meaning of human coitus with what they view as degrading animal copulation." Rock denied any reasonableness or merit in prolonged marital continence, a practice propounded by the Church when a mother's health or family distress made the prospect of more children dangerous. Rock questioned whether for the vast majority of married couples, "this is not for them an unnatural, and if so, a sinful practice." Short-term continence, he allowed, is usual in practically all cultures, possible, useful, and clearly harmless. As a contraceptive measure, however, he cautioned it was far from reliable.

While the major thrust of his lecture concerned population control and the "now urgently required restriction of births," his equally impassioned message was for understanding the good use of sex. "Only by the good use of sex," he emphasized, "can Man escape stress and insure the survival of his kind so that healthy, educated descendants may grow in wisdom."

In correspondence during this period with his bountiful benefactress, Mrs. Katherine McCormick, he indicated how well aware he was of the risks he was taking. In one note, he wrote, "I find myself more than ever in the forefront of the gradually increasing efforts of many to weaken the traditional opposition of my Church's officials to rational methods of birth control. An exceedingly frank statement of wherein I believe they are wrong will be broadcast by the New York station WBAI tonight. This, together with my recent publications, is bound to advance me to the firing line, if not to the wall." Rock had his own definition for the ingredients of a good speech: "A good speech consists of a good beginning and a good end, in close proximity. Like a washing machine, after it spins itself dry it should shut itself off, automatically."

At an appearance at Ohio University, he asked: "Why do we fool ourselves into thinking that adequate food supplies [in the face of a ballooning world population] will prevent the destruction of civilization? There is no doubt that the earth could theoretically support many more human beings. But, we know now that food is not enough for survival, not to mention happiness. . . . [Like overcrowded animals who first turn on one another and then become impotent] perhaps that is our future: That we breed ourselves first into irrationality and then sterility. As Sir Julian Huxley has said, 'It has become wrong and indeed immoral to put obstacles in the way of bringing the rate of increase down, as Roman Catholics, puritans, fundamentalists, Marxists, and other frightened, dogmatic or reactionary groups have been doing.' It hurts me to have to say that he is right. Let those in high ecclesiastical places face what is already a fact of life in many parts of the world: Distraught parents taking the only step available to them in the absence of proper instruction in and equipment for the practice of birth control. They are destroying before they are born, nearly one-half of their conceptions. If these escapes be immoral, how much more immoral is it to make this the only alternative to utterly unnatural and unacceptable [sexual] continence?"

A few days after the assassination of President John Kennedy on November 22, 1963, Mrs. McCormick wrote to Rock saying: "I have taken the catastrophe very hard. He was the best of us — you know — we are not likely to see as good again." Rock wrote back to her: "I feel exactly as you do — sunk. But we have got to carry on. I give a lecture in London on Monday, one in Amsterdam on the following Thursday and home to speak at the Ford Hall Forum in Boston on the 15th [of December 1963]. I hope I am doing some good."

In another lecture, Rock recalled being asked by a young medical student, "What is the most dependable contraceptive?" Rock replied, "The same as it always was — fifteen feet of fresh air." Rather than being facetious, he used the ancedote as a springboard for pressing home the point that birth control methods had to be acceptable. "Continence," he said, "except between two saintly partners — and they are few — weakens marriage and that is bad for mankind." He also noted the futile efforts by Gandhi in India, "where ascetic denial of the flesh has long enjoyed a prestige rarely attained in the Western world" to exhort couples to practice continence in marriage. "Overwhelmingly clear," Rock said, "is the fact that not in Boston, nor Bombay, nor anywhere between those areas are there more than a microscopic few, who could achieve this saintly triumph over sex, and but an inconsequential few more who would want to do so." It was cultural naïveté and outright stupidity, he said, to try to induce women in India to accept rhythm as a birth control method, as was tried in one WHO experiment. Strings of colored beads were given to women who neither had calendars nor were able to read them if they did. The beads were of two colors, "red" for the days in the menstrual cycle when the women were likely to be fertile and should "stop" having intercourse, and "green" for the sterile days when they could "go" ahead. Only later was it realized that the Indian culture permitted coitus only in the dark. Different shapes then were substituted for the "safe" and "unsafe" days, but then it was discovered that the women believed the mere wearing of the beads protected them. Any acceptable method of contraception, Rock instructed, had to be humane, had to have wide applicability, and had to be reversible. It also could not disturb any other bodily system or function. "In parts of Africa," he pointed out, "a man will discard his wife if menstruation fails. Thus, we see that our compulsion to restrict conception is no easy matter."

On a stage at the Boston Museum of Science, shared with the British social commentator Alistair Cooke, a population watcher by avocation, Rock recalled an encounter that occurred in São Paulo, Brazil, while he was speaking to a national Catholic physicians congress. He had sat beside a very pretty, thirty-five-year-old Canadian nun-nurse, while a Parisian physician named Dr. Chauchard discoursed on intramarital continence. "The French doctor, somewhat to my surprise," Rock said, "insisted that a properly loving couple could relatively easily refrain from all sex relations, even for a prolonged period of time, if necessary. In a proper state of love, Dr. Chauchard said, it was perfectly reasonable to think they could share the same house, bedroom, even the same bed, without difficulty, while forgoing all sexual relations. He said it could be done in the same spirit of love in which brother and sister live together, without sexual temptation. I asked the nun if she believed this. She smilingly, and I think rather diffidently, said, 'Yes, of course. It is what we are taught.' Then, I asked her, why did not all the priests and nuns live together in the same convent or monastery in the same loving brotherly and sisterly manner without fear of any intimacy? She merely roared with laughter and gave me no answer. I dubbed Dr. Chauchard, Father Chauchard; I think somewhat to his discomfiture."

It was with such needling stories that Rock most tellingly irritated Church conservatives. They considered such jibes both irrelevant and irreverent. Rock knew better. He knew they really hit home. Such stories carried on the wind, were remembered and repeated and enjoyed. Best of all, while people were laughing over them, the point sank in and made people think.

Between 1960 and 1965, when the papal commission held its first meeting, usage of the pill in the United States had grown tenfold, from fewer than five hundred thousand women to more than five million. In the intervening years, the pill found many critics, had prompted congressional hearings, and had led the Federal Food and Drug Administration to advise that the pill not be used for more than two consecutive years until further studies could be made. Much of the concern was spawned by early reports, primarily from Great Britain, that some women developed abnormal blood clots while using the pill, causing some to have paralyzing strokes or heart attacks. A few deaths resulted from these pill-associated consequences. Moreover, some women found other far less serious side effects to be unbearable, such as nausea, weight gain, swelling of the feet and hands, and a peculiar "tanning" of the skin around the eyes. Such symptoms of course are all also associated with pregnancy, the condition the pill mimicked. Not all pregnant women experience the symptoms, nor did all women taking the pill. The estimates were crude, but the incidence of the side effects was said to be between 10 and 15 percent; about the same number as in the original Puerto Rico studies.

To investigate the seriousness of pill side effects, the FDA created a task force on the subject, comprised of members of the agency's Advisory Committee on Obstetrics and Gynecology. In 1966, the FDA report was filed, an extensive document that explored every alleged adverse effect of the pill. The importance of the study was obvious. "The oral contraceptives present society with problems unique in the history of human therapeutics. Never will so many people have taken such potent drugs voluntarily over such a protracted period for an objective other than for the control of disease. These compounds, furthermore, furnish almost completely effective contraception, for the first time available to the medically indigent as well as the socially privileged. These factors render the usual standards for safety and surveillance inadequate. Probably no substance, even common table salt, and certainly no effective drug can be taken over a long period of time without some risk, albeit minimal. There will always be a sensitive individual who may react adversely to any drug and the oral contraceptives cannot be made free of such adverse potentials. The potential dangers must be carefully balanced against the health and social benefits that effective contraceptives provide for the individual woman and society," the report noted.

The Task Force particularly examined three worrisome possible adverse affects: thromboembolic (blood-clotting) disease, cancer potential, and diabetes. To deprive a large population of drugs of great benefit by overattention to adverse effects based on animal data, the task force said, was unjustifiable. While various types of adverse experience were discussed, the report emphasized that "most of them occur naturally, with a definite though low incidence in our population." The task force also noted the hazards in assumptions regarding cause and effect between any drug and an adverse effect. They often are coincidental. Nonetheless, the task force stressed the need to know how safe the pill really was. Conceding that the information available was not really sufficient (neither in this study, nor in the early British studies, was any attention paid the relationship of smoking to pill-associated side effects; later studies in the 1970s found smoking to be the most important contributing factor in raising the risk of blood-clotting in pill users), the task force in general found that the risk of blood clots was extremely low; the time of use was too short to evaluate cancer promotion potential, but if the oral contraceptives were cancer causing "they cannot be very potent"; and the diabetic or other glandular effects closely correlated with pregnancy itself, tending to be more visible during pregnancy and regressing after pregnancy (or pill usage) ended. The task force recommended large case studies of pill users; long-term followup; continued surveillance of pill use; uniformity in reporting suspected adverse effects and in labeling of the various forms of the pill; and allowing lower doses (strengths down from the original 10 milligrams to 5 and 2.5 milligrams; today, 1 milligram strength mini-pills, only one-tenth the original dosage, are available) of the pill to come on the market with less red tape. But the most significant recommendation of the task force was to lift any ban on length of pill use. "There is no scientific justification for the present restrictions. They are often circumvented and serve only to penalize the large indigent populations." Though the issues of safety would follow the pill through the next fifteen years, at the time in 1966, the FDA's clearance for the pill amounted, in part, to another setback for Rome. Women would not be easily touted off it out of fear for their health and Rome could not retreat into that argument — health protection — as an escape route from confronting the challenge the pill presented.

Just as the pill continued to stand the test of time in the mid-1960s, so did Rock. His status continued to rise and his ideas to take root.

While Rome wrestled with its conscience over approval of birth control, another world institution, Harvard University, decided that the time had come to lend its leadership to attacking the problem of runaway population growth. Under the careful hand of Dr. John Snyder, dean of Harvard's School of Public Health, the university created a Center for Population Studies. Its establishment was founded on the realization "that rising population density threatens to vitiate the gains made by civilization." Also recognized was the conviction that the health profession must now "embrace the consequences: of its success in reducing infant mortality and lowering the death rate of older people the world over." The new center's primary objective was to help amass the knowledge to solve "the immediate task confronting civilization . . . to achieve a sharp reduction in birth rates in many parts of the world."

To get the center started, Snyder first set up a new department of "Demography and Human Ecology." He needed a chaired professorship to kick it off. The announcement of the new center was made at a meeting of the Associated Harvard Clubs held in Cleveland. A few days beforehand, Snyder sent a copy of the text of his announcement to John Rock. While in Cleveland Snyder received a phone call from Rock, saying he thought the center was a great idea and that he wanted to help in any way. "He said he'd come to see me," Snyder recalled, "that he had some ideas. The best one was that we go to see John Searle [president of G. D. Searle and Co.]." Snyder wrote to Searle and got an immediate response. He was open to the idea of funding a chaired professorship, but he wanted more details. "He stated emphatically, that he wanted someone appointed who would be directly involved in human studies, some one directly in the action, not a theoretician," Snyder says. "We arranged to meet on September fifth [1963] at his Chicago office. John, of course, came with me."

Snyder told Searle that he had clearance from Harvard that a chair would be acceptable in the name of John G. Searle or any member of his family. Further, Harvard would be amenable to a ten-year payment plan for the professorship. (The price then was $400,000. Today a million-dollar endowment is required.) Searle had a better idea. He proposed to give $50,000 a year personally and $50,000 more from the Searle Company for four years — or possibly less time, if a merger with the Abbott Company worked out well. Then, Searle stated his conditions. He wanted no mention of the Searle name in connection with the gift. He wanted to have the chair named the John Rock Professorship. "The naming of the chair for John came as a complete surprise. He was very much moved. He got up and walked around the room — tears came to his eyes. He spoke up after a few moments to say that there might be objection or reluctance on Harvard's part because of his book and because of the next book that he had in mind. He felt because he was Catholic and controversial there might be difficulties for Harvard. I assured both Searle and Rock that Harvard was very proud of him and that in my opinion Harvard would be pleased to honor an illustrious emeritus professor, without worry over possible criticism stemming from religious sources. Mr. Searle seemed pleased." Harvard, of course, was delighted. Such magnanimous gifts were not easily come by in those years any more than they are today.

Three years later, in 1966, Harvard conferred its highest honor on Rock, awarding him an honorary degree. At the graduation ceremonies he was named honorary Doctor of Laws in the same company with dancer-choreographer Martha Graham, poet and critic Mark Van Doren, and artist and sculptor Alexander Calder. The degree carried the inscription: "To thousands of grateful patients he has given the joy of children; to millions of families the potentiality of a happier life." For Rock it was an undreamed-of reward. He loved Harvard with a fierce loyalty, second only to his Church.

Meanwhile, a new entry in the contraceptive field made its debut — the intrauterine device, or IUD. Actually it was an old idea with a new twist. In past centuries, Arab camel drivers had placed pebbles in the wombs of the animals to prevent pregnancy during long journeys across the desert. In the mid-1800s, a variety of "stem pessaries" were developed, consisting of a tube inserted in the vaginal canal and fitted with a button that anchored the tube outside the cervix. Improperly handled, they caused terrible pelvic infections. As James Reed pointed out in *From Private Vice to Public Virtue,* these early IUDs became the "symbol of the suffering sure to follow attempts to thwart nature's law and society's rule by separating sex from procreation." Early in this century, however, a German gynecologist, Ernst Grafenberg, developed a true IUD, made of silk gut and wire, that he tested in one thousand patients with a high degree of safety and effectiveness as a contraceptive. Others, less fastidious than Grafenberg, had far poorer results and the IUDs again fell into disrepute for good reason. Pelvic infections were dangerous and frequently deadly before the era of antibiotics. All this, however, preceded the discovery of plastics. In 1958, a Berlin-trained obstetrician, Lazar C. Marguilies, on the staff of Mt. Sinai Hospital, New York, came to Alan Guttmacher, chief of obstetrics there and an adviser to the Population Council. Marguilies had an idea for an IUD made of molded plastics. Its great advantage was that though it was shaped like a coil, it could be stretched out straight for insertion and then, inside the womb, it would spring back to its coiled form. It meant the IUD could be inserted without the painful procedure of dilating the cervix. Although Gutmacher had warned against IUDs, in his popular marriage manual, he allowed Marguilies to test the delicate, lightweight, and best of all, inexpensive new devices. They worked far, far better than their crude prototypes, although some women expelled them and others experienced painful cramping and excessive menstrual bleeding. The Population Council invested more than $2.5 million in clinical trials of the new IUDs. By 1967 family planning programs in South Korea, Taiwan, and Pakistan, which relied heavily on IUD use, began to have an impact on birth rates.

Marguilies said he'd been inspired to try to develop a workable IUD after he heard John Rock lecture on the dangers of overpopulation. Rock never warmed up to the IUD method; never prescribed one. He distrusted the long-term safety of maintaining an irritant, which the IUDs were, in the lining of the womb. Twenty years later, Rock's concerns were largely vindicated as troublesome chronic pelvic infections became widely associated with long-term IUD use.

Within the circles of population control agencies, the arrival of the IUD provides hints of the halfhearted support they originally gave the pill. In the early 1960s, representatives of the Population Council frequently made veiled references to the "commercial interests" behind the pill. Long after preference studies showed that women here and in developing countries favored the pill over the IUD, the Population Council lagged behind in including the pill in its family planning programs.

The availability of the pill (and later the IUD) also changed United States policy on family planning at home and abroad. In 1963, largely at Senator J. William Fulbright's behest, the United States Agency for International Development (AID) was allowed to spend funds "to research the problems of population growth." Senator Ernest Gruening, M.D. (Democrat of Alaska), a long-time birth control crusader, and Senator Joseph S. Clark (Democrat of Pennsylvania) moved to have the National Institutes of Health begin funding contraceptive research. When President Lyndon Johnson's War on Poverty opened in 1964, the new Office of Economic Opportunity was able to fund community groups to undertake domestic family planning programs. The page turned irrevocably with Johnson's 1965 State of the Union speech in which he declared, "I will seek new ways to use our knowledge to help deal with the explosion in world population and the growing scarcity in world resources." It was a new ballgame. Where anti–birth controllers for years had been able to stop the dispensing of contraceptives through public programs on the basis it was an unjustified, if not immoral, use of taxpayers' money, suddenly their arguments no longer held. The new question, in the light of Johnson's War on Hunger overseas and his domestic War on Poverty, became instead, how could the United States justify withholding contraceptive service from the poor, services now readily available to the middle class? The answer was it couldn't be justified. As a result, in 1967, for the first time, AID began funding population control programs abroad, largely operating through private agencies such as the International Planned Parenthood Federation, the Population Council, and the Pathfinder Fund. The same year, the Social Security amendments designated that no less than 6 percent of maternal and child health service funds were to be allocated to family planning. This marked the first time that contraceptive programs were included in federal welfare policy.

However, as the papal Birth Control Commission deliberated on acceptance of the pill, Rome also was confronted by the other "new" method, the IUD, that quickly gained widespread acceptance and support. While the precise mechanism whereby IUDs interfere with conception is still not fully understood, the generally accepted basis is that the IUD, acting as a mild irritant, either prevents a fertilized egg from nesting or alters the motion of the Fallopian tube so that an egg moves more rapidly through its passageway. In the latter instance, an egg would move too quickly for fertilization or there would be insufficient time for a fertilized egg to mature to the point it was prepared for the next step, nesting in the womb. If nesting were in any way interfered with, the Church would view the process as a form of abortion, even though there is no certainty, and certainly no proof in any given month of a woman's cycle, that the IUD is having an abortifacient effect.

Finally, in April 1967, the first break came in the wall of secrecy that had enshrouded the papal commission. In a journalistic coup, the *National Catholic Reporter* obtained and published the first three "working papers" the commission had prepared. The fourth was obtained by the London publishing firm of Burns & Oates in September 1968 and published in England by *The Tablet* and in the United States by the *National Catholic Reporter*. Neither the authenticity nor the accuracy of the reports has ever been disputed. The reports themselves gave strong indications the birth control rule would be changed. What's more, they showed the votes were heavily in that column. Though the exact vote has never been revealed, Father Murphy says, "as far as can be determined, the experts voted for change in the Church's teaching by a majority of some 60 to 4, and the executive committee of cardinals and bishops by nine to six. Thus, the world knew that a substantial majority of the double Commission had recommended liberalization on birth control with a solid theological justification for doing so, and without restricting the contraceptive methods that could be licitly used." *Mirabili dictu,* the commission had voted for the whole package, had approved not only the pill, but virtually the full range of birth control methods. It accepted birth control fully in principle. The wedge driven into the Church's prohibition by the pill, it seemed, might topple the whole wall. In the light of later events, it is worth noting what the various positions of the commission were.

The conservative view is said to have had as its main author the Reverend John Ford, S.J., a Jesuit professor of moral theology at the Catholic University of America, plus two other Jesuits, a French population expert and the Redemptorist Reverend Jan Visser of Rome. The report essentially held that contraception is always a serious evil, *analagous to homicide,* a damnable vice. It held that it was not new teaching on the malice of contraception that was evolving, but new teaching of "sexual concupiscence in the new use of marriage." Sexual relations were said to carry a special inviolability because they generate life. If contraception were approved for the married, the next question would be why not outside of marriage. Approval of contraception would undermine objection to other evils — oral and anal copulation, masturbation, and possibly sterilization and abortion. "Conjugal love requires no specific carnal gesture, much less some determined frequency." Evidence of this was noted in the "intimate love between a father and daughter, a brother and sister, without the necessity of carnal gestures." But above all, the conservatives argued that the Church could not have been wrong about contraception, or else God must be on the side of the Protestants: "If contraception were not intrinsically evil, in honesty it would have to be acknowledged that the Holy Spirit in 1930, in 1951 and 1958 assisted Protestant churches, and that for half a century . . . a great part of the Catholic hierarchy . . . condemned most imprudently, under the pain of eternal punishment, thousands upon thousands of human acts which are now approved. . . . For the Church to have erred so gravely in its responsibility of leading souls would be tantamount to seriously suggesting that the assistance of the Holy Spirit was lacking to her."

The second "working paper," entitled "The Question Is Not Closed," was the liberals' response. It was prepared by Father Joseph Fuchs, S.J., of West Germany, Canon Philippe Delhaye of France, and Father Raymond Sigmond, a Dominican teaching in Rome. It shrugged off the 1931 papal encyclical banning birth control as an understandable reaction to the Protestant approval (at the 1930 Lambeth Conference), and a reaction partly based on the fear at the time that contraceptive practice would undesirably reduce world population. The report contended that sexual acts are the sources of life, not the sex organs themselves. It held there was no difference between acts in a fertile or unfertile time. If it was permissible for a man to use his sex organs to foster love or for procreation, it made no difference which purpose was in effect. Children had rights to a decent life and education. It virtually dismissed rhythm and abstinence as deficient and unfitting. And it stressed that where contraception is neglected, abortions are more numerous.

The third document — which in effect became the fourth and final report, along with a preface and amendments — was the Summary Document on the Morality of Birth Control, together with the Bishops' Word on Pastoral Approaches. This, the ultimate report, was a beautifully expressed, conciliatory message. It linked the well-being of the world to the well-being of marriage and the family. It said that parents should conscientiously decide the number of children to have: "Married people need decent and human means for the regulation of conception." When practiced responsibly, the report said, each and every particular sex act need not be open to fecundity, so long as the marriage was; noting that the way for acceptance of this thinking had been prepared by the acceptance of rhythm. The report urgently called for relevant sex education of couples before marriage and the fostering of the role of women in the context of social evolution. The Bishops' Word went further, holding that married couples were responsible "toward each other first, so they can live a love that leads them to unity." The statement explained that "in the past the Church could not speak other than she did because the problem of birth control did not confront human consciousness in the same way. . . . Let not legitimate modifications be taken as casting doubt on the meaning and value of different attitudes in the past."

The document was a marvel of compromise. It courageously advocated change but with grace and adroit face-saving. Rock could not have done a better job of it himself. It was astonishingly close to the line and language he himself had set forth in his book.

No one was prepared for the extremity of Pope Paul's decision, given in the encyclical *Humanae Vitae* (Of Human Life), when it belatedly came on July 29, 1968. It said *no* to everything the vast majority of the papal commission and his executive board of bishops and cardinals had endorsed. It sounded almost as though they had not existed. It echoed only the severe stance of the conservatives.

Humanae Vitae emphasized the "indisputable" authority of the Pope.

It dismissed the conclusions of the commission as not definitive. It recognized the importance of conjugal love only to then settle back to restating the old prohibitions, if anything more stringently than before. Every sex act must remain open to the transmission of life. Man does not have total "dominion" over his sex organs, because they are God's instruments for new life. Rhythm was still permissible — for serious reasons only. Sexual abstinence to avoid pregnancy was proof of "honest love." Among the consequences of contraception were marital infidelity and the prospect that husbands "growing used to contraceptive practices, may lose respect for the woman." Governments could force contraception on their people. Couples were urged to acquire "perfect self-mastery." Only one reference obliquely noted that treatments (meaning use of the pill) were still permissible when "truly necessary." This reference was later shown to be a last-minute insertion.

Many reports pointed to Cardinal Alfredo Ottavani, the head of the Holy Office, as the inner Vatican manipulator who influenced Pope Paul to close the door on birth control. Speaking, as Ottavani said he did, as the eleventh of twelve children, "the freedom granted couples by the [Vatican Council] to determine for themselves the number of their children cannot possibly be approved." Ottavani reportedly gave his own statement (as a member of the birth control commission) to the pope, a statement said to knowingly and cunningly appeal to Paul's characteristic support of previous popes' positions. What Paul VI had done was to reaffirm tradition simply because it is what the Church had always taught.

He was not prepared, however, for what happened. For the first time in papal history, the laity and the clergy simply ignored what he said. For millions of Catholic couples, the papal ruling was shocking. They recoiled in disbelief. They had waited so long only to have their hopes, they felt, betrayed. In Washington, D.C., the very next day, some forty young priests signed a statement addressed to William Cardinal O'Boyle, but publicly released, saying they would not enforce the pope's decision. O'Boyle, though he had been a leader in school desegregation, redrew the old line on birth control, as the pope had directed. O'Boyle silenced and defrocked twenty-five of the objectors, eventually forcing them out of the ministry, seemingly to set an example for Catholic clergy nationwide as to what their fate would be if they disobeyed. Yet, O'Boyle's neighbor, Cardinal Lawrence Shehan of Baltimore, faced with a similar rejection of the encyclical by a number of his priests, did not even press them for a retraction. Almost nowhere, however, was the encyclical received with the "joyful docility" the pope had requested. It was the first encyclical to be openly rejected.

In the United States, within forty-eight hours, a protest statement was drafted by faculty from the Catholic University of America, and eventually signed by six hundred members of Catholic college faculties worldwide. The statement centered on the right of Catholics to dissent from noninfallible teachings. But the bishops of the United States officially endorsed the encyclical and ruled the laity must accept it.

One of the most ardent supporters of the encyclical was the then archbishop John Wright, later elevated to cardinal and head of the Vatican Office for the Clergy. Wright said, "What Pope Paul has done, what he had to do, is recall to a generation that does not like the word, the fact that sin exists; [and] that artificial contraception is objectively sinful."

One of the bitterest critiques came from the late Dr. Andrew Hellegers, a professor of obstetrics at Georgetown University School of Medicine and a member of the papal commission. He called the conclusions of the encyclical disastrous. "It is difficult to see why the Papal Commission should have been called at all," Hellegers said. In essence, Hellegers said the pope dismissed all new information on reproduction, sexuality, and contraception *because they lead to new conclusions.* Logistically, Hellegers said, the pope's stance on rhythm was ludicrous: if rhythm were to be the only method available to Catholics, there were not enough physicians to teach the technique to Catholics, and the doctors were in precisely the opposite place. Geographically, "where the need would be greatest, physicians would be fewest." Hellegers chided the pope for urging scientists to improve the rhythm method. How could that square up, he asked, how would the morality differ between perfect contraception and perfect rhythm?

Other laymen, including non-Catholics, independently took on the pope and the encyclical. Biologist J. J. W. Baker of Wesleyan University, in a scathing review,* cast Pope Paul's reign in population units of time. From the day Paul became pope to the day he appointed the birth control commission, the world's population increased by sixty-three million people, equal to the nation of Nigeria. By October 1965, when Pope Paul spoke before the UN and referred to birth control as "irrational" the world population had increased by an amount equalling

* "Science, Birth Control and the Roman Catholic Church," published in the Journal *BioScience* in 1970.

East and West Germany combined. By the time Paul issued his encyclical, within the period of his reign alone, the world population grew by a number equal to six United Kingdoms. And ten million persons died of malnutrition. Baker concluded, *"Humanae Vitae is not based upon love, as were statements made in the past by the Church; it is based upon biological ignorance."*

Above all else, neither the Catholic hierarchy or social leaders had reckoned with the sound, native instincts and the capacity to make personal judgments of the common man. Catholics, along with everyone else, took to the pill in overwhelming numbers and with great dispatch. Once they made the decision, there was no turning back. The relief they experienced when the constant threat of pregnancy was lifted from their marital lives and the new joy found in hitherto impossible sexual freedom was not to be given up. They had been moving steadily along those new and precious tracks for eight years by the time Pope Paul unveiled his encyclical. For the first time in Catholic Church history, the rank-and-file of the laity simply ignored one of their Church's pronouncements. They concluded that the pope and celibate clergy didn't know what they were talking about when it came to sex.

"It was too late. They'd already made their decision. It was a peculiar historical thing. The pill came along and the Church hesitated and vacillated, while people were making up their own minds. Had the Church acted more quickly, perhaps the outcome would have been different. But as it was, the people reacted by saying, you're wrong on the pill, maybe you're wrong on a lot of other things," according to Father Greeley. "The clergy did not lag behind the laity, either, in deciding that birth control was all right. The laity and the lower clergy changed in about the same proportion at the same time. The laity practiced birth control, the clergy condoned it, and the hierarchy, eventually, looked the other way." From then to now his opinion polls have continued to bear him out and to document that the papal decision against the pill and all forms of birth control has cost the Church dearly in terms of Catholics turning away from the Church, of clergy leaving their vocations, of a sharp fall off in vocational replacements, and in billions of dollars lost in financial contributions. He thinks it is remarkable that in the aftermath of the encyclical, Pope Paul never pressed further for its acceptance, or took disciplinary action against any clergy who opposed it.

From all indications, the Church not only lost credibility with its own on all issues pertaining to marital sex and birth control, but also with the world insofar as any future deference on contraceptive practices was concerned. Never again did the Roman Catholic position dominate a national or international body, when family planning programs were being implemented. The Church's stance no longer carried convincing weight outside of local settings. Rock's arguments, and those of others largely inspired by him, prevailed from then on in the court of world opinion.

For Rock, the papal rejection was singularly disappointing. He had never doubted that when confronted by "right" information, his Church would do otherwise than come to the "right" conclusion. "The hierarchy has made another terrible mistake," he said upon hearing the news. "They already have lost the fight on birth control, and now they will lose the fight on sterilization and abortion."

11

A BITTER TIME FOR ROCK

THE adverse report from Rome on birth control was not the only blow to befall Rock in 1968. It was but one of three, nearly equal in severity, that together would undo his life. Apart from his family, Rock had three unshakable loyalties: his Church; his school, Harvard; and his instrument for combating unwanted or excessive births, the pill. One by one in 1968, all three seemingly were turned against him.

Only months after Pope Paul VI closed the door ecclesiastically on the pill, Harvard, in the guise of its medical school and its hospitals, which he so long had served, closed the book on him and on his world-famous Rock Clinic. If there is any ground on which Harvard's actions might be defensible, it could only be that those Harvard agents who eased Rock out did not know the sorry state of his finances at the time. When Harvard evicted him from his 77 Glen Road enclave, he was literally broke.

In many ways the world in which Rock had practiced medicine and carried out his research was going out of existence in the late 1960s. While the massive new federal programs Medicare and Medicaid guaranteed long overdue medical care to the elderly and poor, the same programs largely served to dismantle the old system of charity medical care. Rock's overlooking of payment and casual approach to billing went out of style. The era of the solitary figure in the laboratory was passing, too. Research had become supersophisticated, involving scientific teams, elaborate equipment, and large grants of money. Sources of funds shifted from private foundations to the government, primarily the National Institutes of Health and other federal agencies. The rules were far stricter, requiring rigorous cost-accounting and detailed administrative reports. Special Internal Revenue Service exemptions had to be obtained to legalize attractive tax-exempt donations.

Since the mid-1950s, Rock had housed his clinic in a building on the ground of the Free Hospital for Women in Brookline. Mrs. McCormick's money had transformed the original "hovel," as she had called it, into a reasonably up-to-date facility. There was a graceful reception area, doctors' offices, and examining rooms on the first floor, laboratory and research facilities on the second, and a combination records room and library and a couple of spare offices on the third. In Rock's estimation the facility was ideal, though it, too, became increasingly congested due to the steady rise in patients. The larger part of his practice remained trying to help infertile couples, who flocked to the clinic by the score as his fame grew; fame fanned by what some of his envious colleagues called "publicity," news stories concerning the pill and his challenge to the Church. More and more, however, patients also wanted contraceptive counseling.

To accommodate the changes governing research and fund-raising, Rock formally incorporated his practice into the Rock Reproductive Clinic and established a sister foundation to serve as a research arm and a conduit for funds. Both entities were licensed by the IRS as nonprofit organizations with independent boards of trustees. Though he was still extraordinarily robust, still maintaining a driving pace and still shaking off minor physical inconveniences, as he saw them — small heart attacks and bouts with bursitis — he knew that his active years were drawing to a close. He knew it was time to make arrangements for his retirement and for the clinic's continued life. All he wanted for himself was a setting in which he could continue to pursue certain lines of research — the scrotal muff, the role of smells (pheremones) as sexual attractants, and unsolved problems of infertility in men as well as in women. For the clinic he essentially wanted only two things: for Harvard to take over the clinic as a permanent institution and for it to be called, in perpetuity, the Rock Clinic. The conditions upon which those two goals were to be met were simple: Rock was to receive a stipend, so long as he was professionally active, of $30,000 a year, and two long-time members of his staff, Mrs. Menkin and another laboratory assistant, Peteris Lucus, a Slavic immigrant who never obtained his license to practice medicine in this country, were to have job security. Rock felt he had to protect them. They, too, were getting along in years and they were professionally and economically vulnerable.

To this day Rock will not discuss what, specifically, undermined the dream, eventually killing it, but documents and the recollection of some who were privy to the negotiations make it clear that Rock's dreams for the perpetuation of his clinic were doomed from 1966 on. That year, the sister-hospitals, Boston Lying-In, Harvard's obstetrics-teaching unit, and the Free Hospital for Women, the school's gynecology-teaching unit, were merged and renamed the Boston Hospital for Women. As with any set of mergers, bitter power struggles developed as the multiple staffs were commingled.' Rock and his clinic were quickly caught in the cross fire.

Rock, it seems, was guilty of two unforgivable academic sins. He publicly outshone other academic and clinical "stars" at the Lying-In and the Free Hospitals, and his clinic had the lion's share of the patients. At that time, Harvard Medical School was associated with three infertility clinics: one at the Lying-In, one at Peter Bent Brigham Hospital; and Rock's at the Free Hospital. But Rock's clinic attracted 75 percent of the infertility patients. Beyond that, after the patients were treated, counseled or, most likely, operated on, and frequently became pregnant, Rock fastidiously referred them back to their own family doctors or referring specialists. He did not routinely pass them along to colleagues at the other Harvard maternity or gynecology hospitals.

At first, Rock had strong support for his plan to have the Rock Clinic become a permanent Harvard enterprise. The then dean of Harvard Medical School, the late Dr. George Packer Berry, pointed out several instances of historic precedent: the transfer of the New England Peabody Home for Crippled Children into the Peabody Clinic for Crippled Children at Children's Hospital Medical Center; the affiliation of the Judge Baker Guidance Center for emotionally disturbed children with Harvard Medical School; the conversion of the Channing Home for Women with Pulmonary Tuberculosis into the Channing Laboratory, a Harvard research unit at Boston City Hospital; the transformation of the Vincent Memorial Hospital into the gynecology unit at Mass. General Hospital. Dean Berry told the Rock Clinic trustees of Harvard's plan to create a laboratory for human reproduction. To this could be added Rock's clinic and the clinic foundation. "As pioneers in this field the Rock Foundation and the Rock Clinic have served humanity nobly. Now . . . this work can most effectively be moved forward within the stimulating setting of the university," Dean Berry wrote to the Rock Clinic trustees.

Rock also had an ally in Dr. John Snyder, then dean of Harvard's School of Public Health, for whom Rock had interceded with John Searle to obtain the professorship named for Rock. Rock, rather cannily, thought the new faculty position might be used to strengthen the clinic in its future operations. Snyder agreed. "I plan to recommend to the President and Fellows of Harvard that the new John Rock Professor in the Center for Population Studies of the Harvard School of Public Health be appointed as the Medical Director of the Center with the understanding that he may also serve as the Director of the Rock Reproductive Clinic on a part-time basis provided that he and the Trustees of the Clinic wish to make such an arrangement," Snyder wrote in correspondence with Rock. "By means of this arrangement it would be the intent of this School to associate its population work with research, both basic and clinical, on problems of human reproduction." Further, Snyder opined, the mutual relationships between the Population Center, Harvard's teaching hospitals, and the clinic would help assure financial support for the clinic. The arrangement would have fulfilled Rock's fondest hopes for an important role for the clinic in the decades ahead.

With Berry's retirement and the other institutional changes in the mid-1960's, those sources of support were lost. Rock Clinic trustee records show a peculiar and persistent frustration of all their efforts to bring Harvard and Rock to mutually satisfactory terms. Meanwhile, even though the clinic patient load grew, research funds were hard to come by. To keep the research going, Rock repeatedly plowed his own salary back into the work. He kept nearly nothing for himself — only $5,000 to $10,000 out of a designated "salary" of $30,000 a year.

While holding out one hand in negotiations whereby Harvard would acquire the clinic on terms acceptable to Rock, with the other hand administrative factions at Harvard began to squeeze the clinic's lifeline of operations. First, the hospital discontinued support for any residencies or research fellows — always doing so, of course, on technicalities, defendable in principle. Yet, everyone knew that Rock could not function without the manpower the young doctors and fellows provided. Undaunted, Rock raised the money independently for some fellowships and paid a stipend out of his own pocket to others who wished to study under him.

One of Rock's assistants was a young research fellow, Elliot Rivo, now an obstetrician-gynecologist at Newton-Wellesley Hospital in Massachusetts. Rivo was not yet board certified in his specialty during his years with Rock, but he was able, hardworking, exceedingly conscientious, openly ambitious, and unswervingly loyal to Rock. He also was irritated by his exclusion from the high-level discussions over the future of the clinic, and understandably so, since his own future was at stake. At the height of the deliberations, however, Rivo received his draft notice for induction into the U.S. Army. It would have been a simple matter for Harvard Medical School to have Rivo deferred, as he asked to have done. Rock pleaded with the Harvard hierarchy to intervene. He desperately needed Rivo's help with the case load of patients the clinic was carrying. Rock pointed out that in World War I, he had not been released for military service by Harvard. For no stated reason, Harvard declined in Rivo's case.

Harvard kept up the pressure in other ways, too. To an extent never used before, Harvard fussed about egress doors and safety standards. Rock, it must be said, made matters worse through his own doing. He sometimes let Mrs. Menkin and her handicapped daughter, Lucy, live upstairs in the clinic for short periods, when landlords elsewhere made life hard for them. The same Harvard functionaries, however, who rode hard on the Menkins' overnight use of the clinic seemed blind to the fact that during the last years of the clinic, Rock, himself, was living there. They certainly did not bother to find out why.

During the final years that he owned a home in Brookline, he had occupied third-floor rooms as an apartment for himself, renting out the main portion of the house downstairs. Even that, however, became too much for him to manage and he sold the property. He'd always held the family homes in his wife's and, later, his daughters' names, as a protection against lawsuits. When the Brookline home was sold, he shared the proceeds with his daughters. One of them bought a farmhouse in Temple, New Hampshire, which he often used weekends as a retreat house. The arrangement, of course, left him without a home base in Boston. He really couldn't afford to rent, and so he made do with a stark little room up under the eaves in the clinic building. Odd pieces of tubular furniture outfitted the room and he slept on a cot. Rock was a consummately proud man and never let friends or colleagues know the abject state of his finances. Because he kept up appearances, lunching weekly at the Tavern Club and attending the private dinner meetings of the Medical Exchange and Aesculapian Clubs, his secret was well kept.

For nearly three years, discussions among Rock, his clinic and foundation trustees, and Harvard Medical School officials turned on who would be his successor as head of the clinic. The trustees favored Dr. Hilton A. Salhanick, the Frederick Lee Hisaw Professor of Reproductive Physiology at Harvard School of Public Health. Salhanick, who had resigned as director of the Beth Israel Hospital to be free to concentrate on research at the Harvard School of Public Health, really didn't want the job of running a clinic — not even the Rock Clinic. He did then, and still does, however, have a major research interest in the development of new contraceptives. Salhanick genuinely tried to solve the Rock Clinic dilemma and recommended Dr. Janet McArthur, a noted Mass. General Hospital internist-endocrinologist and a distinguished researcher in gynecology and reproductive physiology. At the time, she was a new trustee of the Rock Clinic. Dr. McArthur was not approved. "The Harvard group opposed her for three reasons," Salhanick says. "She was not a surgeon and the clinic practice was strongly surgically oriented; they were hesitant to appoint someone from the 'outside,' and MGH was considered outside the Affiliated orbit; and they were uncomfortable with appointing a woman. Everyone knew what a superb professional Janet was, but that was not the basis for this decision. It also would have meant giving her tenure and a full professorship. No woman at Harvard Medical School or the School of Public Health had ever had that up to that time. Even though some of us on the search committee and Dr. Howard Ulfelder, chief of gynecology at Mass. General [Hospital], supported her, she never had a chance." Although Rock eminently respected and personally admired her, he did not support her candidacy either. He knew that any woman was destined to fail — and the clinic with her — in the ruling all-male "club" at Harvard. In Salhanick's view what really killed the Rock Clinic was "that there was competition for his patients who were essentially private patients and others on the ward service. They felt that by not helping him, the clinic would die and the other two Harvard infertility clinics would inherit his following."

Dr. John Freyman (now president of the National Fund for Medical Education, based in Hartford, Connecticut) was the relatively new director of the merged Boston Hospital for Women during the critical final phase. "Everyone's memory is conveniently fuzzy about it now," he says, "but the heart of the problem at the time was getting rid of Rock. We just have been the best of friends — always — and in our meetings about the clinic, there was no rancor. It just was an untenable situation. It fell to my responsibility as director of the hospital to sit down with him and get him out. He was an absolutely delightful person, sweeping in, wearing an ascot and smoking a curved pipe. But trying to pin him down was like trying to catch an eel. He would have made a superb diplomat. The Free Hospital and Lying-In were merging and it was time to tidy up the clinic's relationship to the hospital. No, it was more than that. The Free had been a tight little island, an incredibly insular little group. They lived in their own world, running their own little preserve. But they were making money hand over fist. The hospital had a huge endowment and a gynecology hospital with all of its surgery is a money machine anyway. Getting rid of Rock was part of the whole endeavor to bring the Free fully into the orbit of Harvard's teaching hospitals. It was a very sad episode. Rock was not reimbursing the hospital for the [clinic] space, not in any realistic sense. He was sort of 'squatting' in the little building across the street from the Free. He had a very large clientele, a lot of patients. But the clinic itself had no real substance, academically. He had a couple of really marginal people on his staff, Mrs. Menkin and some Eastern European man. We wanted to get rid of them and he insisted they had to stay on the payroll. He wanted the clinic under the wing of Harvard Medical School, but he would not part with the name. He was not about to step aside and not see his name perpetuated. As I remember it there was some kind of a deadline. We needed the revenue [from Rock's patients] and we needed the space. No, it really wasn't the space. We just had to get Rock out of there."

At one point, Miss Grahn and Dr. Freyman offered Rock the alternative of moving his clinic into the basement of the Lying-In Hospital. The space they had in mind were the long-since-abandoned nurses' live-in quarters. They were dark, cramped, dismal, and decrepit. Rock wanted no part of them. He'd gone through enough turmoil getting the 77 Glen Road facilities renovated. What was being offered was in worse shape to start with and, though he was assured the space would be "fixed up," they all knew the struggle involved. Money for extensive renovations wasn't available and Rock, intuitively, distrusted a relocation into the Lying-In building; he sensed that "his" clinic would rapidly become "theirs."

The *coup de grâce* came in a 1967 memo written by Dr. Charles Easterday, one of a four-man ad hoc committee from the Boston Hospital for Women who sifted the options for the final disposition of the Rock Clinic. Some of the "insiders" on the scene at the time ascribe a

touch of Brutus to the memo. Easterday had been one of Rock's pro-
tégés and had moved on to become an understudy* to the late Dr.
Duncan Reid, the masterful chief of staff at the Boston Hospital for
Women and holder of both the William Lambert Richardson professorship in obstetrics and the Kate Macy Ladd professorship of obstetrics and gynecology at Harvard Medical School. On the committee
with Easterday were Reid, Dr. Freyman, the hospital director, and his
assistant, Gerald Mungerson. Easterday's memo expressed, it is said,
what Reid and Freyman wanted. The solution, according to the memo,
was basically to take over the clinic and further to expand it, excluding
Rock entirely. Easterday wrote "the Rock Clinic should be voted out
of existence except in name only. (It is my firm belief that it will slowly
'die on the vine' without further financial support and guidance.)" He
adjudged the space in the clinic (space Mrs. McCormick, of course,
had renovated) to be "somewhat extravagant." It could be condensed,
making room for an additional chief-of-staff. Easterday also recommended that a residency program be set up, rotating residents, fellows,
and postgraduates through the clinic; just as Rock had wanted but was
denied. Easterday thought that if the infertility clinics at the Free Hospital and Peter Bent Brigham were combined with Rock's it would
support reproductive surgery on "all days of the week." Easterday also
formulated the rationale that would justify ending Rock's presence and
firing his staff: a "private" clinic was out of place in the Harvard-
hospital sphere and "until the staff is employed university full-time, the
Clinic should not be tolerated."

It took another year to carry it off. By the end of 1966 Rock was
officially evicted from the Glen Road premises. The clinic that had
been his primary professional base and had become his only mainstay
was shut down. His pension from Harvard paid him $75 a year. Ironi-
cally, the clinic was legally dissolved at the hand of Elliot Richardson,
then Attorney General of Massachusetts, who as a young man had first
met Rock aboard Elliot's uncle Henry Shattuck's yacht on their once-
a-summer holiday outing. (Elliot and his brother George, an MGH
gynecologist, as teenagers had been mesmerized by Rock when he unabashedly would apply pancake makeup to his face to protect his
supersensitive skin from sunburn. "He knew that makeup was the best
sunshield, but we didn't," George says. Rock also indulged in skinny-
dipping, again, he said, because a bathing suit chafed his skin. "He

---

* In 1971, Easterday became acting chief of staff upon Reid's retirement.

was completely unflappable," George recalls.) The court records show that when the clinic was liquidated, the corporation owed Rock tens of thousands of dollars in back salary, more than the net worth of the entire clinic operation. The final document states that "John Rock has agreed that he will carry on the objectives of the Clinic."

The problem was he had no place to do it, absolutely no place to turn and no one to turn to. Margaret Sanger had died of leukemia in Tucson, Arizona, in September 1966, shortly before her eighty-seventh birthday. Gregory Pincus died tragically in August 1967 when he was only sixty-four years old, of a rare blood disease, myeloid metaplasia, that was said to be associated with his exposure to chemicals used in his research. And Katherine Dexter McCormick's death came in Boston four months later in December 1967. She was ninety-two.

Dr. Robert Ebert, now president of the Milbank Foundation in New York, had barely taken over the reins as dean of Harvard Medical School in 1965 when the move to oust Rock was under way. Ebert was too new to the position, too unfamiliar with the medical politics of the matter, to act decisively at the time. "I was a great admirer of John Rock. He was a very strong personality and very deprecating in terms of his accomplishments. No one could have been less arrogant about what he had done, which I've always felt was the mark of a really important man. He always was a generous man. He delivered our daughter Betsy, when I was an intern at Boston City Hospital. We were referred to him as the best obstetrician in the city. Of course, he never charged us for his services. He never charged any of the interns." Ebert, today, is appalled at the way Rock was treated at the end. "This was a great tragedy. It was a time of great change and egos were all riding high. Rock was well along in age. In those times there was really no arrangement for retirement. People were retired with no pension at all, particularly from the medical school, because they weren't paid through the university." On its own, the medical school, however, often found a place where faculty retirees could continue to work — albeit on a less physically taxing schedule. As an example, Ebert cited Arthur Hertig, Rock's long-time research colleague. "Arthur Hertig retired with practically no pension. That's why we gave him the job at the primate center out in Westborough. . . . He was very competent and besides, he didn't have enough to retire on. The same is true of several others."

No one in all of the Harvard hierarchy, however, found a protected corner in which Rock could go on with his work. He was on his own.

In January 1969, finances forced Rock to sell his practice and the prized name of the Rock Clinic. It was purchased by a young colleague, Dr. John H. Derry of Newton, who established the Rock-Derry Clinic and took over all but a single office in the professional suite at the edge of Roxbury, where Rock had attempted to relocate the clinic. It was a standard purchase and sale. Rock agreed to end his practice and turn all his women patients over to Derry. All Rock could legally continue to do was pursue research activities, and in a very limited way, lacking funds and without a laboratory. Rock was to be paid for a period of five years, 10 percent of that portion of Derry's net income which exceeded $15,000. Rock's share never amounted to much. For all intents and purposes, the Rock Clinic was no more.

Under these circumstances, it was more than unusual that the Searle Company should quite unexpectedly place Rock on a lifetime research grant. He would continue to evaluate data on the pill for them and carry out other contraceptive investigations of interest to him — and them, indirectly. In return, he would receive a research consultant stipend of $12,000 a year. It was virtually his only income. While it was only a marginal amount to live on, he found it sufficient. He could still pursue his clinical research interest in fertility problems, particularly those caused by low sperm counts in men. He also could and did continue to write philosophic medical essays about population control, when asked, for specialty publications and to prepare lectures for guest appearances at medical gatherings. He never questioned, nor did he have any cause to, the regular check for $3,000 that came four times a year from Searle.

Nonetheless Rock's financial plight was beginning to be whispered about in some of the best places, the Tavern Club and at prestigious medical society gatherings. Monsignor Lally says he heard vague suggestions that Rock was having a hard time, so did Ebert, so did Rock's surrogate sons Luigi Mastroianni and Celso-Ramon Garcia, all the way down in Philadelphia. Lally and Ebert were dismayed to later discover that they didn't really know how bad things were. Both men were certain that Rock's friends would have swiftly and discreetly come to his aid. "Why, when I think of how much money he raised at the Tavern Club for the Free Hospital, and then they just put him out . . . well, that's disgraceful," Lally raged. Ebert echoed the same sentiment. Mastroianni and Garcia, however, from their vantage point as former fellows of Rock's, had very clear insight into how little Rock always had financially taken out of the clinic. They were sure, as soon as they heard, that the rumors were true. They made arrangements for Rock to join them at the University of Pennsylvania, to serve as a kind of elder statesman in their reproductive and gynecology studies. They wanted him as a role model for their students of the ideally understanding and considerate physician dealing with troubled infertile patients, just as he had been a role model for the two of them. Rock, reading between the lines of their invitation to join them in Philadelphia, knew there was more kindness than professionalism in the gesture. He said if he were younger he'd like nothing better, but they should find someone with a more certain future for the job. From Searle's standpoint, there was a little conscience-easing in the move, too. Searle not only had made millions on the pill, but also the windfall had come at a critical time in the company's expansion. Beyond adding to the financial dividends, the pill did a lot to solidify Searle's pharmaceutical stature.

As if the demise of his clinic and the Church's refusal to approve birth control were not more than disastrous enough in 1968 to break his spirit, that year Rock also saw his pill subjected to serious scientific assault. The pill always had its discreditors and, in truth, the pill did cause side effects in some women; in a very minuscule percentage there were serious and even deadly consequences. Dr. Hilton Salhanick, who lent his support to Rock's fight to keep the clinic alive at Harvard, was, in his own words, "a scientific purist at the time." He was intellectually disgusted with the workings and report of a 1965 World Health Conference on the pill held in Geneva. The meeting largely divided into two camps, according to Salhanick, "those who wanted to tout the pill as the greatest thing since cracked wheat or those who wanted it discarded as lethal. A few of the people there wanted a third line of thinking adopted . . . that enough was not known about the metabolic effects* of the pill. That was my position."

Under a grant from the Center for Population Research of the National Institute of Child Health and Human Development, Salhanick organized a prestigious meeting on the pill, precisely on its "multiple systemic metabolic effects"; aspects of the pill he felt had been neglected. Since six million American women were using the pill in 1968, he thought "it was timely and important to examine the biological

---

* Metabolism is the sum total of chemical processes whereby living systems maintain themselves. In the above usage, the term is used to include all the possible chemical effects of the pill on blood, tissue and glands as its hormonal components are processed by a woman's body.

effects" of the pill from a strict research standpoint. So many studies of the pill were taking place that Salhanick (and two associates) were able quickly to assemble fifty-five separate reports on virtually every conceivable physical impact of the pill. The meeting took place in Boston during the first five days of December 1968.

By that time, eighteen variations of the pill were on the market. At the conference, Salhanick stressed that "contraceptive drugs are not 'equal' . . . biochemically, physiologically, pharmacologically or psychologically." Nor, he said, were the synthetic steroids that comprised the various pills natural substances. They behaved differently one from the other, and in a biochemical sense they could not be equated with pregnancy or pseudo-pregnancy. He concluded, however, that despite the extensive reports presented at the meeting "our fund of knowledge [about the pill] is meager . . . more work must be done and new information gathered." Repeatedly, throughout the compendium of the reports, the scientists themselves noted that their data were insufficient, their conclusions tentative, and their extrapolations from animal studies uncertain, in terms of how relevant they were to human assimilation of the pill.

One report stands out, in retrospect. In a review of the pill's effects on the blood and circulatory system, the eminent British epidemiologists Richard Doll and Martin Vessey casually noted: "In our data there was a *suggestion* that women who used oral contraceptives smoked more heavily than women who did not." The physician-scientists noted that "this might account" for some of the instances — rare instances — in which the pill had been related to blood-clotting and other circulatory disorders. In no study reported up to this time had any investigators even looked into the relationship — later clearly established — between the heightened risk of blood clots in pill users and *smoking*. By later lights, the oversight was astonishing.

Looking back, Salhanick now says that his 1968 conference on the pill was never intended as an anti-pill forum. Yet, that is how it was reported to the lay public and how it was widely perceived by the medical community. National medical news writers from across the country wrote story after story, usually topped by scare headlines, about the newly reported hazards of the pill. No organ of the body was unaffected by pill usage, the stories ran; nor was the psyche spared its deleterious effects. Few stories gave equal space to the benefits of the pill that also were reported at Salhanick's conference. "I just was trying to get at the facts, the measurable, provable, reproducible facts about the pill," Salhanick recalled. "I felt then and do now that the truth ought to be known. Yet, there's no denying the conference opened a Pandora's box."

In a completely unexpected way, the timing of Salhanick's conference coincided with the resurgence of the feminist movement in America. Suddenly, the pill, which two of the most ardent feminists of all time, Sanger and McCormick, had ordered specifically so that control of fertility could be placed in the hands of women, became a target of the most militant factions within the new women's movement. By far the most outspoken critic of the pill was Barbara Seaman, a New York medical news writer and columnist for the *Ladies' Home Journal* and *Family Circle* magazines. In 1969 she published her first book, drawing extensively from Salhanick's conference, entitled *The Doctors' Case Against the Pill*. Seaman contended the "one essential book that every pill-prescribing doctor should have" was the compendium of the proceedings of Salhanick's conference. The findings, she held, "were grim." With unrelieved intensity, she stressed only the worst possible effects of the pill, as she has continued to do in the intervening years. Her 1969 book, the first all-out attack on the pill, was instrumental in provoking a round of congressional hearings in Washington, D.C., in 1970, and in stimulating the federal Food and Drug Administration to make drug companies insert a warning label into all packages of the pill. She later co-founded the National Women's Health Network, which apart from its objective of focusing attention on sexist medical practices, also serves as a rallying point for her campaigns against the pill.

Although in the early years Salhanick was not a strong pill advocate, he nonetheless considers Seaman's reporting of the conference biased, and her stance against the pill irrational. "She persists in it," he says, "beyond reasonableness. She's wrong about it. The metabolic problems associated with the pill are not very important when cast against the risk of pregnancy or the alternative of abortion. The pill was and is amazingly safe in light of the numbers that have been used. All of life is a balance between the risks and benefits. I disagree with people who see only the risks. My conference was never meant to be an indictment. At the time it simply represented a forum on the questions and a guide to work on the pill that had to be done."

Salhanick's recollection of the conference seems far mellower today than his action appeared to be at the time. Rock took it very personally. He was insulted that he had not been asked to participate. The conference was held only a few city blocks from his stopgap office in the Back Bay Towers. He disagreed with most of the questions raised about the pill's safety, but neither he nor anyone else had the kind of evidence needed to refute detractors on unassailable scientific terms. Only his experience and his trained instinct kept him convinced that the hazards were grossly exaggerated. The combination of setbacks took its toll. He had less and less physical and financial reserves to call into play. In March of 1970 he was eighty years old. More and more frequently, he retreated for long weekends to the pleasant farmhouse his daughter had purchased in Temple, New Hampshire. He kept going until 1971. Then, his relationship with Dr. Derry grew sour, and finally the day came when he had to tell Mrs. Menkin he could no longer employ her. There was nothing left to pay her salary. Rock moved the few worldly possessions that he treasured up to Temple: his books, his diaries, his pictures . . . of his wife Anna, his son Jack, his daughters and his grandchildren. It was time to sit back and let the rest of the world catch up with him.

As the decade of the 1960s closed, eight to ten million American women were taking the pill daily, despite the often exaggerated headlines of pill-associated health hazards. There also was wide acceptance of all forms of birth control. One by one, the state laws prohibiting or limiting birth control or the use of public funds to pay for contraception for indigent women had come off the books.

As late as 1964, however — four years after the pill was federally approved and being taken daily by millions of American women — seventeen states still regulated or prohibited outright the advertising of contraceptives or the sale of condoms by vending machines. Eight states still prohibited the sale of contraceptives by licensed pharmacists or physicians, two states prohibited their sale but permitted doctors to prescribe them, and two states prohibited their sale but permitted the sale of medical works describing contraceptive methods.

Connecticut went farther than any other by making it a criminal misdemeanor to "use any drug, medicinal article or instrument for the purpose of preventing conception." As *Time* magazine reported in 1961, "Late every night in Connecticut lights go out in the cities and towns, and citizens by the tens of thousands proceed zestfully to break the law."

In Massachusetts, where anti–birth control laws were bemusedly codified under a section delineating crimes against chastity, it was not illegal to *use* contraceptives, as it was in Connecticut. Little else was exempt, however. It was a felony to exhibit, sell, prescribe, or provide contraceptives, and though rarely enforced, to disseminate birth control information.

It did not escape John Rock's attention that "it must have amused some of the citizens of the Commonwealth of Massachusetts, with its rigid law against birth control, to discover that the first breakthrough in contraceptive technology in seventy-five years suffered and survived its labor pains in the environs of Worcester and Boston. Life, indeed," he noted, "has a way now and then of mocking man's more questionable designs."

Massachusetts had liberalized its anti–birth control statute in 1967, largely through campaigns led by Drs. Duncan Reid and David Rutstein of Harvard Medical School and Dr. Joseph Dorsey, a young Catholic doctor in training at the Peter Bent Brigham Hospital, and by Edward Collins, a member of the faculty at Boston College, the oldest Jesuit university in North America. Predictably, however, Massachusetts could be counted upon to make one last-ditch stand. It enacted a statute that still prohibited the dispensing of birth control materials to unmarried women, a measure immediately challenged by the self-styled birth control and later abortion crusader William Baird. In March of 1972, the United States Supreme Court declared that act discriminatory and unconstitutional. In striking it, the last anti–birth control law in the United States was finally off the books.

In the court of public opinion, the pill still held sway. Even the pill's severest critic Barbara Seaman, acknowledged that "the pill remains attractive to women for two important reasons. Except for the word 'no,' it is the most effective and convenient reversible contraceptive ever devised. No wonder Margaret Sanger lusted for it, and no wonder other liberated women have agreed with Clare Boothe Luce that with the pill 'modern woman is at last free, as a man is free, to dispose of her own body, to earn her living, to pursue the improvement of her mind, to try a successful career.' "

12

THE PILL COMES OF AGE

> The pill, in time, will usher in the golden age of womanhood. It will set them free as nothing before in history has. It will enable them to plan not just for their pregnancies, but their lives. Employers will not be able to shut women out of important jobs any longer on the ruse that an unexpected pregnancy might interefere with its completion. Women will be able to pursue higher education and higher professional goals. They also will be free to spend more time with the few babies they do have. It [the pill] also will set their husbands free. They will not be crushed under the burden of supporting large families, locked into jobs they hate but can't afford to leave and overwhelmed by the responsibilities of trying to be a good father to a house full of children. More than all that, the pill will do something absolutely transcendant for the world. It will usher in the age of the wanted child. Just think of it, every baby wanted, loved, held to be precious and dear, provided for and nurtured! The pill will not do all this by itself, but by also gaining acceptance for all forms of birth control. But it is the pill that will be the lever for change of a magnitude none of us has dreamed possible.

So said Dr. Andrew Elia in 1965 when he was chairman of obstetrics and gynecology at Boston University School of Medicine.

That year some five and a half million American women were using the pill; consuming sixty-five million cycles of it. In 1981, the year that the pill came into its majority — became twenty-one years old — an estimated billion cycles of the pill were marketed worldwide; some sixty to seventy million women were relying on its contraceptive power.

While the pill and other contraceptives have not yet brought into being the golden times that Dr. Elia foresaw, the pill indeed has wrought colossal social change in the still very short time it has been available. "It changed the world. There's no doubt about it," said Dr. Louis Tyrer, medical director of the Planned Parenthood Federation of America. "The great social changes of the past generation are largely based on the contraceptive movement. And in the future, contraception is going to spread more and more across the world. After just two decades of use, oral contraceptives are today the most popular reversible method of contraception in the world."

Here in the United States, where the pill was born, its impact is at least partially measurable. It came into being just as the stirrings of renaissance were reawakening the feminist movement. "For the population that was college age when the pill was introduced, it was the flagship which led the subsequent flotilla of 'women's liberation.' The pill became a central part of the educated young woman's existence in the 1960s," Elaine M. Wolfson, Ph.D., of New York University's graduate Public Administration faculty pointed out. Composite forces were at work she noted, "but the chain of events and the profundity of its impact placed the pill in the position of being one of the major antecedents of the women's movement. The coincidence was monumental."

Women not only have gained greater freedom to work but they also have been able to enter careers that previously were the province of men. In 1960, 32,000 women were in the military; in 1980 there were nearly 150,000. Moreover, the number who were officers has doubled. In 1960, a mere 387 women became medical doctors out of 7,032 M.D.s awarded that year; by 1980 nearly 3,000 women received their M.D.s, about one-fifth of the total class. "Probably, the largest change has taken place in the numbers and rates of women training in the law," Professor Wolfson went on. Only 230 women graduated law school in 1960 out of a total of 7,657, but by 1980, nearly 9,000 did, approximately one-fourth of the graduating class. Beyond the professions, women overall have moved into the work force in unprecedented numbers. In 1960, only 37 percent of American women of reproductive age were employed. Today, 60 percent are, and the number rises each year.

In a talk entitled "Effects of the Oral Contraceptive and its Meaning for Women" delivered at the first Annual John Rock, M.D., Commemorative Symposium, University of Pennsylvania School of Medicine, October 21, 1980, Professor Wolfson stressed that "one final perspective should be added. As a result of the oral contraceptive, women have acquired virtually the same rights with regard to pregnancy and sexual activity that men have always enjoyed. Since 1960, a woman is able to make a unilateral contraceptive decision without obtaining the cooperation of her partner. Until that point only men enjoyed such latitude. It is this autonomy in reproductive matters that is crucial to the development and manifestation of rational self-interest [by women]. And without such rational self-interest, freedom and responsibility are only a charade. In my judgment, the oral contraceptive has probably done more for equal rights for women than any other single phenomenon."

Other drastically different societal patterns also have come about as a ripple-effect of the pill and its consequent, nearly universal, acceptance of birth control. The marriage age has risen. Where 28 percent of women in the twenty- to twenty-four-year-old range were single in 1960, nearly 50 percent are unmarried today. The "desired" number of children has dropped. In the mid-1960s, only one to two percent of women eighteen to thirty years old expected to have no children, while 30 to 35 percent of them expected to have four or more. Today, approximately six percent of those under thirty signify they want no children, the vast majority want only two, and only seven percent envision having four or more. The actual birth rate in the United States dropped from 24 per thousand of the population to a low of 14 (the rate has rebounded to 17 in early 1980 — due to the number of women in their thirties who are having their first — delayed — pregnancy). In twenty years, the United States has achieved nearly zero population growth. A seldom-recognized boon has been the availability of birth control to low-income and minority women. In the mid-1960s only 17 percent of American black women in their most fertile years (fifteen through thirty-four) were using the pill, largely because birth control was not covered by welfare or other public health facilities. Today, nearly twice that number are using the oral contraceptives.

One of the great ironies in the twenty-year history of pill usage in this country was the extent to which it was attacked by a minority segment within the women's movement. In his book *The Politics of Contraception,* Dr. Carl Djerassi describes them as "a radical fringe of well-meaning, affluent, middle-class members of some women's rights movements . . . seemingly without any awareness of how culture-bound their

arguments are." The anti-pill faction insists that women have been un-
fairly — unilaterally — saddled with responsibility for birth control,
as well as being subject to dreadful hazards from the pill. Barbara Seaman summarized in large measure their stance in testimony before the
House Select Committee on Population in Washington, D.C., held in
March 1978. She said: "Many of us are willing to return to the 1950s
contraceptive technologies (essentially, the condom and diaphragm,
and even rhythm methods) and make them work, but we are not being
well served by today's physicians and clinics." That view, however, has
relevance only for highly motivated women with strong educational
and economic resources. For them, multiple choices of contraception
are reasonable, even if not fully reliable. A physician herself, Dr. Tyrer
of the Planned Parenthood of America is a classic example of how
traditional modes of contraception can fail even in expert hands. "I
had eight pregnancies while using the diaphragm," she said. Djerassi
further points out, "The diaphragm may be ideal for the motivated
American women willing to use it, but it is totally unsuitable for the
impoverished woman living in a hovel lacking running water, toilet
and privacy. The reality is that for many women throughout the world,
the pill is the best contraceptive method currently available. It is this
last factor that is ignored totally by some feminists and by many other
affluent, middle-class Americans." Frederick Jaffe, president of the
Alan Guttmacher Institute, also has countered the anti-pill arguments.
Speaking at the Women's Center of the University of California, in
1977, he said: "Two of the most profound social changes of the last
twenty years have been the increasingly more effective regulation of
fertility and the widespread movement for altering the roles and status
of women. . . . Both of these processes have been facilitated . . . by the
emergence of a new contraceptive technology based primarily on the
oral contraceptive." Insofar as substituting other methods for the pill
are concerned, he said, "It is a particularly class-bound assumption,
which ignores the difficulties low-income women had with traditional
contraceptives before the advent of the pill and their quite different experience with it. Those who advocate replacing the pill with a diaphragm, the condom or other coitally related methods may be speaking
for themselves, but . . . they are not addressing the needs of the bulk
of low-income women in the U.S."

Even more surely, American feminists who oppose the pill on the
idealistic ground that it makes life riskier for impoverished women in
Third World countries simply miss the point. It is one unwanted preg-

nancy after another, imposed on top of chronic hunger and abject want, that beats such women down. While well-intentioned American feminists *want* the right thing for their deprived sisters — contraceptive choice and a sharing of contraceptive responsibility by both husband and wife — the gap between the ideal and the possible is too great. Of what use to millions of Asian women are diaphragms, when they are homeless, migrating from one feeding camp to another, lacking water to drink, never mind to clean diaphragms. Even in better circumstances, cultural and religious taboos preclude any likelihood that they can use traditional contraceptives. In many Eastern cultures, touching one's genitals is forbidden as is allowing a male doctor to demonstrate how a diaphragm is inserted or for him to insert an intrauterine device (IUD). Men, in most of the countries with the largest populations and lowest economic wealth, are culturally adverse to using condoms. While the IUD is the cheapest, reversible contraceptive, it has built-in disadvantages as a contraceptive for women in underdeveloped countries, even where there are no religious barriers. A trained health worker must be available to insert it, and IUD use often causes pelvic inflammatory disease that requires further medical care. Moreover, women using IUDs tend to have a far heavier menstrual flow and greater blood loss. The resultant anemia is a serious health matter for women already weakened by malnourishment and prolonged breast-feeding. For them, contrary to the case for well-fed American women, the pill is a health boon since it protects against anemia by reducing monthly blood flow by as much as 80 percent.

Despite protestations by Catholic advocates of natural family planning (a more refined version of the rhythm method) that the method is reliable and can be taught on a huge scale to semiliterate and illiterate people, the evidence does not stand up. Though Catholic-sponsored studies contend otherwise, repeated efforts by organizations such as the World Health Organization to initiate natural family planning programs have consistently failed. Rarely can more than 5 percent of the group of potential users be recruited to take part in the program. Because the method requires the support and cooperation of the husband and sexual abstinence during a portion of each month, the method has little attraction for people whose lives have little other comfort in them. Even among highly motivated couples, the failure rate using natural family planning is about 20 percent.

Of all the methods of contraception now available, the one that has gained the greatest universal acceptance is sterilization. In countries as diverse as the United States, China, India and Mexico, sterilization is equally accepted. Puerto Rico and the United States now stand at the top of the scale with one-third of all women who have ever married, now permanently sterilized. In general, where sterilization and the pill are equally available, twice as many people of child-bearing age are now sterilized as use the pill, the second most popular method. Today, worldwide, more than 100 million people — far more men than women — have undergone tubal ligation or vasectomy. And the trend is for sterilization at increasingly younger ages, now often before the age of 35 in developed countries and before 30 in Third World countries, where marriage and child-bearing are customary in the late teens. One reason, of course, why the numbers of the sterilized are so high is that the figures are accumulative; once sterilized, always sterilized. Pill use rises more slowly because as some women begin to use the pill, others stop; collectively, then, there is a constant shift in the body of users.

No one knows for certain how many abortions are performed yearly, worldwide, but the best international estimate is 40 million. Although abortion now is legal in all but a few dozen countries, the lack of public funding for abortion means that millions of women still undergo back-alley abortions every year with devastating effects. In some sections of India, until recent years, abortion carried a 50 percent mortality rate; in Bangladesh, the abortion death rate still is as high as one in three in rural areas. Regardless of the risk, desperate women continue to seek abortions as they always have. Arguments against abortion propounded by well-meaning pro-life advocates rarely recognize the deadly implications of outlawing abortion. In Rumania, for example, when the government became concerned about the rapid drop-off in the birth rate, very restrictive abortion laws were enacted. As a result, deaths from abortion skyrocketed from fewer than 50 per year to more than 300 a year. In countries where abortions are legal and sound medical practices are enforced, the death rate from abortion during the first eight weeks of pregnancy is so low it is barely discernible, less than one in 100,000 women. Even late-stage abortions carry a death rate of less than 2 per 100,000 under optimum conditions. Most reproductive specialists view abortion as a contraceptive failure. Abortion should be preventable. The ultimate goal of good contraceptive practice is to reduce the need for induced abortion to an absolute minimum. Until contraception is universally available, however, abortion in many countries is used as a direct means of birth control, such as Japan. As Djerassi pointed out, "When an estimated eight percent of the world's fertile women undergo abortion in a given year," irrespective of religion, economic status or location, "then it is all too tragically obvious, that unmet contraceptive needs still exist on a vast scale."

Although pill use is now rapidly increasing in Asia and Latin America its use has leveled off in Western Europe and declined somewhat in the United States. This has largely resulted from the growing popularity of early sterilization and from widespread media reports of hazards associated with pill use. Since 1970, the pill has had an almost unrelieved bad press in the United States.

The first wave of the attack came with a series of hearings between January and March 1970 before Senator Gaylord Nelson's Subcommittee on Monopoly of the Select Committee on Small Business. Before they ended, testimony filled three volumes totaling 1,402 pages. Coverage by the national press was intensive. Newspapers given to sensationalism ran headlines about the "Wave of Alarm over the Pill." National columnist Jack Anderson wrote that he had "uncovered a new and frightening danger" — youngsters poisoned by the hundreds from inadvertently taking their mothers' oral contraceptive pills. Anderson's story derived from testimony by one of John Rock's old enemies, Dr. Herbert Ratner, a state public health commissioner, who testified that child poisoning from the pill had "a high incidence in the United States." Ratner, Anderson, and the rest of the American press failed to report the scientific data on the matter, which had been printed five years earlier, showing that when children accidentally swallowed the pill, it had no lethal effect. In contrast to two hundred deaths a year from aspirin poisoning in children, no child has ever died or been seriously sick from inadvertently swallowing birth control pills. Day after day, the hearings, often on the basis of personal anecdotes, thrust before the American public unqualifiedly terrifying accounts of blood clots, heart attacks, hypertension, diabetes, loss of ear wax, liver tumors, potential cancers, loss of sex drive (or worse, increased sex drive), gall bladder disease, migraine headaches, and mental depression.

Little to no attention was paid the testimony of Dr. Elizabeth Connell, then a professor of obstetrics and gynecology at Columbia University and now associate director for health services at the Rockefeller Foundation. She testified, in part: "Virtually nothing has been presented in these hearings that those of us working in the field have not heard many times over. It has frequently been asserted that the hearings, thus far, have been slanted, one-sided and unfair. What I think is needed is a better look at the vast majority of women who can and are taking oral contraceptives safely and effectively.

"As a physician," she testified, "who began to practice before the advent of the pill, I am constantly aware of the immense difference it has made to the lives of women, to their families and to society as a whole. The look of horror on the face of a 12-year-old girl when you confirm her fears of pregnancy, the sound of a woman's voice cursing her newborn and unwanted child as she lies on the delivery table; the absolutely hopeless feeling that comes over you as you watch a woman die following a criminal abortion; the hideous responsibility of informing a husband and children that their wife and mother has just died in childbirth — all of these situations are deeply engraved on our memories, never to be forgotten. . . . The thought that we may once again be forced to face these disasters on an increasing scale because of the panic induced by these hearings strikes horror into the hearts of all of us who have lived through this era once before."

Little attention also was paid to the fact that two years before the Nelson committee hearings began, three large studies, aimed at evaluating the benefits and risks of oral contraception, were started, two in the United Kingdom and one in the United States. The first of these investigations was the Royal College of General Practitioners (RCGP) Oral Contraceptive Study. It involved some 46,000 women, recruited and followed by 1,400 general practitioners. Most of the women are still under observation. The second, the Oxford Family Planning Association (Oxford FPA) Contraceptive Study enlisted 17,000 women attending seventeen large family centers. This study also is continuing. The third study, the only major American study, involved 16,500 women who were members of the Kaiser Foundation Health Plan in northern California. Because they joined the study by having a general health check-up in an automated multitest laboratory at Walnut Creek, it became known as the Walnut Creek Contraceptive Drug Study. It issued its final report in 1981 and has ended because further funding was denied.

As the preliminary reports from the British studies began to appear, however, once again the headlines, particularly in the United States, screamed about the pill's serious side effects. The major problem was a higher risk of dying from a cardiovascular — heart or circulatory — disease. The first RCGP study estimated the *relative* risk of death from a cardiovascular disease was four times greater among women who used the pill than among those who did not. The problem, which has persisted, with the study was that it was based on statistical extrapolations from only twenty-four actual cardiovascular deaths linked to pill use. Further, the rates included women with conditions conducive to circulatory system diseases as well as women with no such condition. The Royal College study also showed the risk was not the same for all women. Age, smoking, and the length of time on the pill all greatly affected the risk of death. More than all else, the study disclosed the dangerous connection between smoking and taking the pill.

The preliminary findings of the Oxford FPA study, published at the same time, reported far fewer deaths, but the distribution of mortality seemed to bear out some of the Royal College findings. In summary, in the larger British study (the RCGP study) pill users' rates of deaths from circulatory disease were estimated to be relatively high — about 40 per 100,000 woman-years of observations — for smokers and women over 35; and much lower (under 15 per 100,000) for non-smokers and women under 35. In the smaller Oxford FPA study, seven out of nine of the actual deaths were among women who smoked and seven of the nine women were thirty-five or older. In that study, there were no circulatory-disease deaths among nonsmokers under thirty-five. Second-stage reports from the British studies held that the findings were virtually the same in twenty-one countries beyond Great Britain. These suggested that such mortality risks were to be found wherever the pill was used.

In 1979, two major reports challenged the death rate associated with pill use, as estimated in the British studies. The first report by Dr. Christopher Tietze, a distinguished biostatistician with the Population Council in New York, was entitled "Where Are the Deaths?" Tietze pointed out that death due to cardiovascular disease in the United States had been declining steadily among women (and men) of reproductive age since 1950. And even more importantly, that the decline since the arrival of the pill had been steeper for women in each age group than for men. If the pill were truly a high-risk factor for cardiovascular disease in women, how could the death rate be going down? Since the smoking habits of women had become similar to male habits in the same period, Tietze said, it would have been expected that women's cardiovascular risks would have risen. While he felt that pill use may increase a woman's risk of *some* cardiovascular-disease death, he felt that the risk would be more likely to be associated with age, smoking, and obesity. "The level of risk attributed to the pill," he concluded, "appears to be exaggerated." The second study was directed by Dr. Mark A. Belsey, in the Human Reproduction Program at the World Health Organization in Geneva. Belsey's study reexamined the British reports that said the higher cardiovascular-disease death rates prevailed in twenty-one countries studied, and presumably everywhere the pill was used. Belsey's reanalysis failed to find any such thing. He found little to no relationship between pill use and higher mortality trends on a world scale. "Given the striking differences in life-style, environment, and physical form among women in the various parts of the developing world and women in developed countries," Belsey cautioned, "it is clearly not prudent to transfer findings from one setting to another."

On the occasion of the pill's twentieth birthday, a benchmark for a medicine in massive use for two decades, a spate of reports reassessed the pill anew. Consistently, the pill was found to be safer than early studies suggested. Further, there was increasing evidence that the pill was protective against some of the very disorders, such as cancer, that it originally had been feared the pill might cause.

One report, "The Pill at 20: An Assessment," was prepared by Drs. Howard W. Ory, chief of the epidemiologic studies branch, Family Planning Evaluation Division of the federal Center for Disease Control, in Atlanta, and Allan Rosenfield, director of the Center for Population and Family Health and professor of obstetrics and gynecology at Columbia University. Noting the intense scrutiny to which pill use has been subject, "studies involving hundreds of thousands of women," Ory and Rosenfield said, "we can conclude with some assurance that for most healthy, young women, the benefits of oral contraceptive use continue to outweigh the risks." To properly evaluate the pill, they said, it must be viewed in the perspective of risks associated with pill use and risks associated with pregnancy and/or other forms of contraception: "As previously noted [in 1979 and 1974 studies], annual pill-associated mortality in the United States is 3.7 per 100,000 users, ranging from 1.8 for non-smokers to 6.5 for smokers. The U.S. material mortality rate is about 20.6 per 100,000 live births — or more than five times higher." For developing-world women, pill use would save many lives, Ory and Rosenfield pointed out, since their maternity death rate is as high as 250 to 1,000 deaths per 100,000 live births.

In October 1980, the final report of the ten-year $8.6 million Walnut Creek Contraceptive Drug Study, funded by the National Institutes of Health and directed by Dr. Savitri Ramcharan, also was complete. "The main conclusion from this study is that in a U.S. population of young, adult, healthy, white, middle-class women, the risks of OC [oral contraceptive] use are negligible." For the first time, a major, long-term study of thousands of pill users found that the users, rather than the pill itself, were the critical culprits in pill-associated disorders. Ramcharan found pill hazards were related to smoking, alcohol use, exposure to sun, and sexual activity.* When the influence of those factors were accounted for the study concluded:

• There is no evidence of an increase risk of cancer of the breast, endometrium (uterus), or ovary associated with pill use. Conversely, pill users have less nonmalignant cystic disease of the breast.

• Pill use in itself does not increase the risk of cancer of the cervix, as had been suggested. But it was common to some oral contraceptive users in the study to have intercourse at a young age and multiple sex partners, two factors long known to be related to cervical cancer. The difference in sexual activity between pill users and nonusers accounted for the difference in risk of cervical cancer.

• There is no increase in risk from circulatory disease among pill users who do not smoke . . . regardless of age. However, when heavy smoking and pill use were combined, they compounded the risk of circulatory diseases.

• An increased risk of malignant melanoma (a serious cancer) of the skin was associated with oral contraceptive users of all ages in the study. However, the researchers also found that the participants in the study all had a significantly higher exposure to sunlight, a factor which has been previously linked to skin cancer among pill users compared to nonusers.

In yet another report on two decades of the pill, Dr. Theodore King, director of Obstetrics and Gynecology at Johns Hopkins University School of Medicine in Baltimore, Maryland, stressed the point that the pill in use today has changed drastically from the first pill marketed. The net result is that earlier long-term studies of oral contraceptives are probably no longer relevant.† Pills commonly prescribed in the early 1960s contained approximately three times the amount of estro-

---

* The population studied was almost exclusively Californian or West Coast women. The women tended to be taller, thinner, blonder, physically and sexually active, well organized, moderate drinkers, and sunbathers.

† The most recent RCGP study showed no cases of arterial disease among users of the lowest dose pills.

gen and ten to twenty times more progestin than the pills prescribed today. A variety of studies have confirmed that lower estrogen doses have decreased the risk of blood clots in veins and arteries.* New reports also have suggested an explanation for the synergistic relationship between smoking and pill use in setting the stage for heart attacks — though it should be emphasized the heart attack risk is extremely low. The reason may be a link between the effects of smoking and birth control pills on lipoproteins (fatty acids) used to transport cholesterol through the blood stream. Here, too, the low-dose pills may overcome the problem, for it has been found that they increase a type of fatty acids (high-density lipoproteins) that are protective against high blood cholesterol levels.

Other fears also have been assuaged. There is no evidence that the pill impairs a woman's ability to have a child when she discontinues pill use, as had been alleged, although return of fertility may be temporarily delayed. Pill users enjoy a far lower risk than other women of ectopic pregnancy, and no different risk of miscarriage, a low birthweight or malformed infant, or stillbirth. The two major British studies have found no evidence that pill use increases the risk of diabetes, another widely broadcast charge. Another new study finds no significant association between the pill and urinary infections. While some studies report an increase in mental depression among pill users, others report an increased sense of well-being. There is no consensus on emotional effects. The twofold increased risk of gallbladder disease among pill users reported in the 1970s has been completely refuted, although this risk had been widely accepted. A benign (noncancerous) tumor of the liver that had been linked to the pill has been shown to occur only in rare circumstances (1 to 3 cases per 100,000 users) and in women who have been long-term (more than five years) users of the old-style high-dose pills. But perhaps the most reassuring news about the pill relates to cancer. It is now conclusive that the pill does not cause breast cancer, and further, there is strong evidence that the pill protects against ovarian and uterine cancer.

In the prevailing news climate of English-speaking countries, where press coverage tends to magnify the negative, scant heed was paid to

* Many others agree with King. Ory and Rosenfield, for example, also state that "most of what we know about the pill concerns formulations used in the late 1960s and early 1970s; these tended to have higher doses of estrogens than do pills today. Thus, findings from earlier studies may overstate the risks to women in 1980."

the well-established health benefits of the pill. The twenty-year assess-
ments emphasized this discrepancy. Women who take the pill are one-
fourth as likely to develop benign breast disease as nonusers. They
are one-fourteenth as likely to develop ovarian cysts. They are two-
thirds as likely to develop iron deficiency anemia, and they are one-
half as likely to develop rheumatoid arthritis. "Since these conditions
are common," Ory and Rosenfield point out, "this reduced incidence
is a very real bonus." The ripple effect of these protective aspects of the
pill is that among every 100,000 pill users there are some 270 fewer
surgical procedures performed for ovarian cysts and benign breast
disease. Pelvic inflammatory disease, a common, serious infection
known to be a major cause of infertility and ectopic pregnancy, also is
reduced. Pill users appear to have only half the risk of this disease,
according to a recent report. Protection against pelvic inflammatory
disease, Ory and Rosenfield contend, "may well be one of the most important noncontraceptive benefits of the pill." Almost never mentioned
is the pill's prevention of dysmenorrhea — painful menstruation, which
though non–life threatening is the most common cause for absenteeism
from work in women, costing them and their employers millions of dollars and lost work-hours every year.

   Though the risk of blood clots and consequent heart attacks or
strokes is small for pill users — and largely preventable, most scientists
feel if the women do not smoke — for the rare individual who is
stricken, the result is undeniably disastrous. Common sense dictates
that women with any potentially troublesome health factor — hypertension, high cholesterol levels, obesity, diabetes, and over the age of
forty — should avoid use of the pill. Though news reports always speak
in terms of threefold, fourfold, tenfold increases in risk, it should be
borne in mind that the basic incidence of blood clots, heart attacks,
and strokes is small in pre-menopausal women. As a World Health
Organization report pointed out, to put into context a finding of five
times greater mortality in pill users than never users, it means the pill
decreased the chances of survival from 99,995 per 100,000 to 99,974
— a reduction of a negligible two-hundredths of one percent. In view
of these baseline considerations, Ory and Rosenfield feel that "it is
ironic that a decline in pill use in the United States appears to have
occurred among young women, the population at lowest risk of serious
side effects." While Ory and Rosenfield feel the challenge is to com-
municate to women as clearly as possible which of them can use the

pill safely and which cannot, they feel it is unlikely all risks can be eliminated.

What would go a long way to relieve anxieties over the safety of pill use would be a test to identify which women would be likely to develop blood clots if they took the pill. A Duke University scientist, Dr. Salvatore Pizzo, not only feels he has discovered the basis for such a test, but also reports that very simple exercise can overcome the hazard. Pizzo and his colleagues have identified an underlying defect in the blood system that is responsible for breaking down clots. Women who've clotted while on the pill have very low levels of a key protein in the blood-clot-dissolving process; a protein called plasminogen activator or PA. However, exercise dramatically increases levels of the protein, especially in those with the lowest level. Pizzo suggests that all women on the pill begin to exercise. "We found that the amount of releasable PA was four times higher in healthy subjects than the women in the study who had clotted while on the pill," he reported. "While we were doing our pill study, we noticed that a few of the women had fairly high levels of PA. We found exercise was the only thing which differentiated them from everyone else in the study group." Pursuing this lead, he studied volunteers who were entered in an exercise program at the Durham, North Carolina, campus. All of them increased their PA levels and, those with initially low levels of PA showed the most dramatic increase. Most importantly, for protection against pill risks, women showed greater increase in PA levels with exercise than did men. The exercise program was a moderate one, basically ten minutes of stretching followed by thirty minutes of walking or jogging, three times a week. While the Duke study does not expect an inexpensive PA test to be available for several years, "the prudent answer is that exercise would be a reasonable prescription for any woman who's using birth control pills." Beyond its relevance to pill use, Pizzo's findings can be applied to a whole range of clotting problems. The work also sheds light on the issue of heart attack and stroke in general, since other studies document decreased levels of PA in people with heart attacks and stroke.

Perhaps, Pizzo's discovery provides an additional explanation for why women in developing countries do not seem to experience the same degree of serious side effects from the pill as women in industrialized nations. They hardly lack vigorous exercise. There are, however, other equally obvious reasons. Women in underdeveloped areas differ in many ways from their more fortunate sisters: in life-style, genetic heritage, diet, and smoking habits, to name but a few. For whatever reasons, they simply do not share the same cardiovascular disease risks of economically privileged women. The British physician A. G. Shaper has observed that "in the tropics, even the obese, sedentary, severely hypertensive, long-standing diabetic does not (except with the rarest of exceptions) develop coronary artery heart disease." It has long been known that in developing countries the incidence of circulatory system diseases is low (with the occasional exception of hypertension) and many "Western" risk factors are far less prevalent. This suggests a double advantage for developing-country women insofar as pill use is concerned. Women in these countries also tend to have low cholesterol levels. Further, they tend to be nonsmokers.

Overall, the risks of using contraception are far outweighed in developing countries by the far greater risks of pregnancy and childbirth. The women know it. Whenever and wherever contraception have been made available to them, economically deprived women have reached out for birth control. Virtually every current survey of the still unmet need for contraception shows that the demand is rising to an unprecedented extent. A 1979 report of women in São Paulo, Brazil, who were without any means of contraception, showed that 20 percent wanted to delay the next birth, while an astonishing 80 percent wanted no more children. While most socialized countries subsidize family planning, in the United States the cost of each monthly cycle of the pill rose in 1981 to six to ten dollars as a prescription purchase. Through bulk purchasing, a comparable month's supply can be obtained for seventeen cents, which with shipping costs averages twenty-five cents per month's supply. Though the cost seems low by Western standards, it is immense for hundreds of millions of Third World families who struggle to survive on per-capita incomes of a hundred dollars or so a year.

Individual hazards associated with pill use become ludicrous in proportion to the magnitude of the problem in trying to deliver the pill to people who need it. This pill "problem" truly will worsen in the decades ahead. Dr. J. Joseph Speidel of the Office of Population for the U.S. Agency for International Development, has analyzed the future of the pill in terms of funding and distribution. Cast against a projected population increase of two billion people over the next eighteen years (by the year 2000) the outlook is sobering. At present about one-third of eligible couples in developing countries — where 90 percent of the population growth will take place — use contraceptives. The greatest success has been in China, where all forms of contraception are free and available, and the one-child family has been adopted as national policy and is backed by a strong reward-punishment system. If China is left out of the statistics, however, the prevalence of contraception in underdeveloped countries drops to one-fifth of those in reproductive age categories. Moreover, there are vast differences in contraceptive use worldwide, varying from 4 percent in Africa to 40 percent in Asia when China is included. The figure for China alone is 60 percent, where population control has been recognized as the most serious problem the country faces in light of its enormous population of a billion people. To stabilize population in economically disadvantaged countries — that is, for the birth rate to equal the death rate — approximately three hundred million additional couples would have to begin to practice birth control immediately. By the year 2000, twice that number would have to do likewise.

That is far more easily said than done. Of the currently estimated one billion dollars spent annually on family planning in developing countries (other than China) about four hundred million comes from donor sources such as the United Nations Family Planning Agency (the United States government contributes about two hundred million dollars a year). But if contraception in these countries must increase from 20 percent of eligible couples to 80 percent, far more than four times more money will be needed. The reason is that the "easiest" countries — those with the best existing infrastructure for birth control dissemination — are already well under way, Speidel has pointed out. "If this target population doubles, as it surely will, by the year 2000, at least eight times the current expenditures will be required," he estimates. "And if inflation continues at its double digit pace, something like thirty-two times the current investment will be necessary." He envisions a minimum investment by outside countries of thirty billion dollars a year to be necessary by the year 2000 and questions whether foreign assistance will supply sufficient money to make contraception available as needed. It is already clear, he says, that it will be impossible to employ the same standards of medical care in the dispensing of oral contraceptives as is required here. Pills will generally have to be available through health workers. In many of the countries, there is only one doctor for ten thousand, a hundred thousand, or in some instances for a million people. He anticipates that the growth of pill use could rise in underdeveloped countries alone to two hundred million users over the next two decades.

Despite the burgeoning of family planning programs and the vast scale of pill use and sterilization, the world's population continues to outpace all efforts to control it. It is incomprehensible to consider how much worse the situation would be today were it not for the arrival of the pill and with it the renewal of interest in birth control. Optimists point to the fact that the population growth rate has begun to dip, dropping now worldwide to a rate of 1.75. But most world population watchers now hew to the view that the time has come to stop talking growth rates and start talking total numbers. Because the majority of the 4.5 billion people in the world today are young — are in the childbearing years — the numbers are still explosive. For every two people on the globe today, there will be three, eighteen years hence.

One of the most effective advocates of population control, Robert McNamara, the recently retired president of the World Bank, maintains that "the most explosive fact" is the desperate condition of most of the world's people. "One-third of mankind today lives in an environment of relative abundance. But two-thirds of mankind — more than two billion individuals — remain entrapped in a cruel web of circumstances. They are caught in the grip of hunger and malnutrition, of high illiteracy and inadequate education, of shrinking opportunity and corrosive poverty. The gap between the rich and poor nations is no longer merely a gap. It is a chasm. On one side are nations of the West that enjoy per capita incomes in the $3,000 to $5,000 range. On the other are nations in Asia and Africa that struggle to survive on per capita incomes of less than $100." He, along with other experts in the field, agrees that "the greatest single obstacle to the economic and social advancement of the majority of the people in the underdeveloped world is rampant population growth." The notion that family-planning programs are sinister plots to coerce poor people into doing something they don't really want to do is absurd, he says. The prevalence of voluntary illegal abortion, he says, should be enough to dispel that fiction.

Statistics show that abortion today is one of the most common methods to limit fertility even though in many countries it is ethically or religiously offensive, illegal, costly, and medically dangerous. In India, each month, as many as a quarter of a million women undergo abortion. Even in highly Catholic Latin American countries, abortion rates are among the highest in the world; in one country the rate is said to be three times the live birth rate, and in another the cause of two out of every five deaths of pregnant women.

The oft-stated idea that family planning leads to family breakdown is another of McNamara's pet peeves. "A single stroll through the slums of any major city in the developing world is enough to dispel that concept. If anything is threatening the fiber of family life, it is the degrading conditions of subsistence survival that one finds in these sprawling camps of packing crates and scrap metal — children on the streets instead of in classrooms; broken men, their pride shattered without work; despondent mothers, often unmarried, unable to cope with exhaustion because of annual pregnancies — these are not the conditions that promote an ethically strong family life. Family planning is not designed to destroy families, it is designed to save them."

That is almost word for word what John Rock said. His intention in offering the pill to the world was first to save the family and after that, the Family of Man.

EPILOGUE

It is 1982 and John Rock is ninety-two years old, still ramrod straight, his six-foot-three frame lean as a pole, his good sense and self-deprecating wit still intact.

He lives a quiet, easygoing life now, befitting a man of his age, in a weather-stained clapboard house on a secluded hillside in Temple, New Hampshire. The house originally had been used as a hunting and fishing retreat by some sportsmen. Rock's daughter Ellie made a few improvements when she and her family lived there at a time when her husband was teaching in a nearby school. But it turned out to be too remote for them. Rock added pine sheathing, and to give himself a first-floor bedroom, he attached a hunter's cabin at one end.

The place suits him. From every window and from a screened porch, where he likes to lean back in an old wrought-iron chair, there's a long view out over distant valleys. In winter, the road is often impassable with snow; and in summer, the countryside is alive with sweet-scented pine and sugar maple. At every season there is a sense of timelessness and peace.

In the good weather, he spends most of his day in or by a natural pool which he and the young companion who stays with Rock, Mike DeLargey, created by damming a freshwater stream that runs through the property's nine acres.

"I just fall in the pool the first thing every morning as long as the water temperature is up to sixty," says Rock. He usually swims nude, a habit he acquired as a boy and indulged for years in Boston as a regular at the L Street Bathhouse in South Boston.

Because his skin is still supersensitive, he doesn't put any clothes on until he goes back to the house in the late afternoon. He keeps an old pair of Bermuda shorts at hand, so he can pull them on if a visitor arrives "so as not to shock their sensibilities." When he finally does dress, it's usually in a gray cotton jumpsuit that doesn't chafe, often worn with an ascot at the neck.

After his swim, he spends the day in a little screened A-frame cabin that Mike built at the side of the pool. "I bring my reading stuff down here and during the really hot days, we have our lunch here." Under the peak of the cabin is a loft with a cot, to which Rock climbs by a ladder for his afternoon nap. Though he gave up cigarettes years ago as a concession to his heart attacks, he still loves his pipe.

Mike markets and cooks for Rock, whom he calls Doc, takes care of the grounds and household repairs, and in general looks out for him. They get along together remarkably well, serving as surrogate father and son to one another. Each time Mike leaves — for school or to do an errand — Rock, mindful of the time his own son Jack left never to return, admonishes: Drive carefully, take your time.

The house, as the plaque given to him by his long-time friend Ben Duffy says, is clean enough to be healthy and dirty enough to be happy. Old habits die hard, however, and though it's been years since he's been inside a laboratory, Rock still carries on his own small studies. He and Mike have tagged certain chipmunks to see how they divide their territories. An ardent birdwatcher, he keeps a log of birds sighted on the property. And he still keeps his diaries, a practice that goes back to boyhood. Last year, as his always difficult handwriting became illegible, he taught himself to typewrite. Three or four times a week, in winter, he goes to a health club in the next town, Milford, for baths in a hot water pool and for massages, the passive exercise he adopted years back after one of his early coronaries.

"I stopped cerebrating at least ten years ago," he is fond of saying. "I can't imagine why anyone stops by." He no longer seeks out the shakers and movers of the world, as he once did, and rarely do they come looking for him anymore, as they once did. Those who come now come out of friendship and admiration. And news reporters still come by occasionally, too, particularly in 1980 for the twentieth anniversary of the pill.

Mastroianni and Gracia make it a point to get up to Temple at least once a year. So do Monsignor Lally and John Snyder, and Ben Duffy makes the trek even more often. Duffy is a special friend, now. He first made Rock's acquaintance in the 1960s, when Rock was already in his seventies and the pill roiled in controversy with the Church — Duffy's church as well as Rock's. They are much alike in many ways and there is a special bond between them. Duffy, too, is a handsome and urbane man, an intellectual Celt and a philosophic Catholic. In earlier years, they also shared a joyous interest in a perfectly chilled martini. Their comradeship goes back to the days when Rock still lived in his Allerton Street, Brookline house. When Duffy would be in Boston, on science excursions while he was still director of the Kennedy Center for Population Studies, which he had co-founded at Georgetown University, he'd always stay with Rock.

Duffy recalls with enormous pleasure nights they spent together, talking until the early hours of the morning. "Then, bright and early, John would be up, playing John Philip Sousa marches on the phonograph, and striding up and down. He said it was a good way to get the circulation going," Duffy says. Now, when he stays with Rock in Temple, Duffy says there's a variation on the ritual. "One February morning, he turned me out of bed shortly after dawn and handed me an old terry-cloth robe — he wore one, too — and a mug of hot tea laced with honey. 'Drink it down,' he said, 'and come with me.' The next thing I knew he had gone out back and thrown himself into the snow, directing me to do likewise. There we were, like two scrawny Don Quixotes, or even more, like crazy old Lear and his Fool, rolling around the snowbank in freezing-cold weather. John told me, it was a perfect way to clear the head. At first, I was petrified because of his frail cardiovascular system, but later, when I stopped to think about it, I realized it was actually very good for the heart. He was creating his own sauna effect. The hot tea and sugar to warm and fuel the system inside, and the cold as an external stimulant. He knew what he was doing." Rock still psychically runs "by his own sense of himself," Duffy holds. "To the very end of the road, he's going to make sure he takes care of himself."

Few people know what an ardent feminist Rock was, in the deepest sense, Duffy feels, or what a total expert he was on human sexuality. "He was enormously interested in women, felt total admiration for them. He was utterly impressed by women, what they could do and how much they were willing to bear. He would often talk to me about how much better women were in genuinely taking care of people.

'Perhaps, it's because they die a little themselves, every month,' he once told me. He saw in the menstrual cycle a life cycle in miniature: the preparation for new life, the readiness, and then the denouement. He also could talk about sex, as a basic biological need, from every aspect. He understood all sides of the phenomenon. He was a walking compendium of sexual knowledge. He went to Kinsey's laboratory and later to Masters and Johnson's and came back rather bemused. He kept pondering the ethics and physiological validity of wiring people up to measure sexual impulses. And it did not escape his notice, that at least in the early years, they used female sex surrogates but not male. In so many ways, as the reports on human sexuality have been published in recent years, it strikes me that they've come now to the level of understanding where John was years ago."

Rock's whole life was exemplified by his courage, Duffy points out. "He took on unpopular causes and when the chips were down, he was out there on the front line almost alone. He also was the inveterate Catholic. It was a hard thing for him to take, after his book came out, the baseless charges that he was promoting scandal or misleading people. Nothing could be further from the truth. It was absolute nonsense. He did not want anything to disrupt his relationship with his Church. He is a very profoundly religious man, fundamentally moving in a Chardin-like movement toward another and another higher level. Once his mind has reached another dimension of understanding, he never goes back to the earlier position. He has made a great difference in my life, but far more than that, he touched the essential chord in every heart."

John Rock is far removed from the hue and cry of the world now, out of the fray. Or almost so. His great disappointment, of course, came with Pope Paul's papal encyclical, that ruled against contraception for Catholics. He still cannot understand the decision. He remains convinced that had Pope John XXIII lived, he would have sanctioned change. What Rock can't fathom is how Pope Paul could have gone to India and South America and personally witnessed the famine and starvation and not changed the rules. In an interview with his journalist nephew, Jerrold Rock Hickey, Rock said, "The last time I was there [in India] I left in despair. Delhi was bad enough. But Bombay was incredible. And I could see no point in continuing on to Calcutta. Pope Paul had been to India, he had seen all the evidence he needed. Yet, he ruled out use of the pill and so far as anyone can tell, he did this individually. The whole process moves so slowly."

Rock still thinks the Catholic hierarchy will one day get around to sanctioning birth control. He was convinced that a new pope would do so in 1978 after Pope Paul VI died. That hope went by the boards with the elevation of John Paul II, the former Cardinal Wojtyla of Krakow. Any doubts about his conservatism regarding sexual issues were quickly dispelled during his historic visit to America in 1979. Repeatedly and in the strongest terms, the pontiff took the opportunity to reiterate official Catholicism's opposition to "the ideology of contraception and contraceptive acts."

When the 1980 World Synod of Bishops convened in Rome to review "The Role of the Christian Family in the World of Today," Rock's hopes flickered briefly again. Speaking for the National Conference of Catholic Bishops of the United States at that meeting, Archbishop John R. Quinn of San Francisco made it clear that birth control remains the thorniest of issues for the Church, the issue that won't go away. "The issue of contraception is an immense problem for the Church today," Quinn said. "Rejection of the Church's teaching on contraception is widespread. In the United States alone nearly 80 percent of Catholic women use contraceptives while only 29 percent of American priests believe that contraception was intrinsically immoral and only 26 percent of priests would deny absolution to those who practice it." Others echoed Quinn's concerns: prelates from India, the Netherlands, Tanzania, England, South Africa. The Redemptorist, Father Francis X. Murphy, writing under his own name rather than his earlier nom de plume, Xavier Rynne, reported in *The Atlantic Monthly,* of the Synod: "The sermon with which Pope John Paul closed the bishops' synod came as a shock. He said the teachings of *Humanae Vitae,* which condemned artificial contraceptives, are incontestably binding. That the Pope chose to ignore statistics pointing to a 2.6 billion population increase by the year 2000 AD hardly seems in keeping with the Church's claim to exercise a catholic care for all the world."

The sociologist and pollster Andrew Greeley simply thinks it no longer matters. "Catholics gave the Church's position serious consideration and they said, no. The whole thing is really sex. The papal decision is that you can stop having children, but you can't have sex. Well that may be a position that some superannuated bureaucrats in the Roman Curia would push who probably don't know the meaning of sexual desires of any kind, but it isn't the position that most parish priests would push. Who is the Church, anyway? If you've got 85 percent of the Catholic laity and all the North Atlantic countries, including daily and weekly communicants, saying contraception is right, then how can it be said the Church is wrong? They're the Church. Maybe some Church authorities are wrong.

"They've simply blown their credibility on sexual matters sky high. They've done it on premarital sex, on abortion, on everything else. One can't find anything in the New Testament to justify their position, one can't find anything in the ancient traditions of the Church. The fact of the matter is that John Rock won. He won going away. John Rock beat the Pope. . . . I can't speak as a moral theologian, I can't judge the matter on that ground. But as a sociologist I can tell unequivocally, Rock won, the Pope lost."

It is all quite immaterial to John Rock now. He has no time to waste on bitterness. Every now and then the world seeks him out again. In 1978, he was honored as an outstanding physician and scientist as part of the Leaders in American Medicine series sponsored by Harvard Medical School and the Countway Medical Library. He came down from his hillside retreat for that. In October 1980, the University of Pennsylvania School of Medicine held the first Annual John Rock Commemorative Symposium, and used it to review the history and meaning of the pill. At the symposium, partly supported by an educational grant from G. D. Searle Company, Rock was awarded a medal in honor of his "research in service of mankind." He reveled in the evening's celebrations in Philadelphia. Little in life could please him more.

Save for these infrequent sojourns, Rock lives now primarily among his memories. He thinks occasionally of the women he helped to have children and those he spared having more children than they wanted. But he says, "I dwell more on the failures. No, I remember those I failed." He regrets terribly that he once — only once — refused a prescription for the pill to an unmarried woman who came to see him. In his own defense, he will only say that his refusal wasn't really due to the fact she was unmarried, but that he was put off by her cavalier attitude about sexual responsibility. His wonderful, strong-boned face still lights up when he is reminded that he was once known as the "saint of Radcliffe."

At first, he doesn't want to countenance questions about whether teenagers should use the pill or whether the pill is the cause of loose sexual morals. Then, he puffs on his pipe and ventures: "I approve of maturity. But maturity is not necessarily chronological. I rather like the acceptance of responsibility which some teenagers are taking. For them, I think it's all right to take the pill. It's better than exposing themselves to a pregnancy. If they are going to play around, they might as well play safely. Premarital sex doesn't hurt most level-headed young people — if they act responsibly." While he concedes that the pill "may have smoothed the wayward path of the young somewhat," he does not for a minute permit the thought that the pill ushered in sexual licentiousness. "If the pill were responsible for that," he retorts, "we wouldn't have so many abortions."

He says he became famous because he had a simple name, just two four-letter words, John Rock. "If my name had been Algernon C. McGillicuddy, none of the notoriety would have happened. It was an easy name for the press — John Rock. I didn't really do very much. I just picked the right concoction, the best one in the lot, right from the beginning."

Today, there are only two things he would like to stress about "this remarkable medication. First, we must remember that oral contraceptives not only can prevent births, but they also can treat various disorders and prevent miscarriage. By preventing repetitive miscarriage, the so-called habitual abortion that plagued many childless couples, the pill has also helped give life. Second, the discovery of the oral contraceptive was truly a team effort. Gregory Pincus and Min-Chueh Chang performed all the complex chemical testing. And Celso-Ramon Garcia and Edris Rice-Wray helped me with the necessary clinical testing of women. I am not the father of oral contraceptives. If anything, I am the stepfather. But as my good friend and colleague Celso Garcia has said, I am the man who put it across, popularized it to a skeptical world."

Rock goes to mass only occasionally now, when there is a funeral or someone is getting married. "I can't follow it anymore," he says. But a crucifix still hangs above his desk.

When visitors come, he receives them formally, with the grace that always has characterized his style. If they arrive on a winter day, he urges them to come into the main room in the house, a book-lined living room where there always is a roaring fire blazing away. With the smoke from his pipe rising around his head, he invites their questions, pausing to turn up his hearing aid. There will be a pitcher of martinis at hand, sitting chilling in the same silver pitcher he used for so many years each evening when he and his Anna had their "quiet" hour. The pitcher was a wedding present.

Along the mantel is an array of photographs, of his daughters, his grandchildren, and his son, Jack. "I can finally look at it," he says, "without weeping if I concentrate on it." His daughters come often to see him now, and he breaks his stays in Temple with frequent visits to their homes. In his bedroom hangs a magnificent portrait of his late wife at the time of their marriage. Her loss still hurts. His eyes fill with tears when he speaks of her death. If memories get too heavy, he goes walking. "I know how to get out of the dumps," he says. "I don't dwell on my losses. I have four daughters, nineteen grandchildren, and now a great-grandchild, all well and happy. And I have the knowledge of the work that I have done. I take a very large dose of equanimity every day, and it works very well." He's sure he's in his second childhood, because his blood pressure is back to absolute normal, "the same as when I was in college."

But John Rock is not a man to delude himself. He looks out over the hills from his hillside vantage point, and he knows the time is not far off when he will pass away. Does he fear death? "I'm too happy with my life for that. I've had six heart attacks and my doctor says I'll drop off in my sleep one of these days. That's all right."

Rather than viewing that prospect with any trace of solemnity, he turns on a full smile and with that irrepressible humor, adds, "So, I just make sure my bed is comfortable."

INDEX

Abbott Company, 183
Abortion, 174, 186; Catholic stand on, 148; spontaneous, 61, 68; worldwide, 213–214, 224–225
Adler, Felix, 40
Adoption, infertility and, 49–50
Adrenal hormones, 102
Advisory Committee on Obstetrics and Gynecology, 181
Aesculapian Club, 197
Agency for International Development (AID), United States, 185, 186, 222
Alan Guttmacher Institute, 211
Albright, Fuller, 101–102
Albright's Prophecy, 101
Albumen, 79
Allen, Willard M., 98–99
American Association of Anatomy, 88
American Catholic Sociological Review, 171
American Gynecological Society, 54, 68
American Society of Clinical Pathologists, 69
American Society for the Study of Sterility, 106, 154
Anderson, Jack, 214
Anglican Church, 25
Annual John Rock Commemorative Symposium, 209–210, 231
Aquinas, St. Thomas, 148, 161
Arnold Arboretum, 19
Artificial insemination, 53
Aschheim, Selmar, 39
Aspiration technique, 48

Associated Press (AP), 69, 85
Association of Large Families (Italy), 159
Atlantic Monthly, The, 230
Augustine, St., 150

Baird, William, 207
Baker, J. J. W., 190–191
Barrett, George, 165–166
Bartlett, Marshall K., 48, 66
Baum, Gregory, 174–175
Becker, John, 150
Bekkers, William, 168
Belsey, Mark A., 217
Berry, George Packer, 70, 87, 195–196
Beth Israel Hospital, 198
Binz, Leo, 176
Birch, Arthur J., 113, 114
Birth Control Commission. *See* Papal Commission on Population, the Family and Natality
Birth Control League (later International Planned Parenthood Federation), 24, 26
Birth control methods: coitus interruptus, 3, 27; condoms, 26, 27, 134, 148; diaphragms, 26, 27, 134, 138, 148, 211, 212; intrauterine device (IUD), 184–186, 212; jellies, 27, 148; rhythm, 26–27, 44, 76, 151, 154–155, 190; *see also* Birth control pill; family planning
Birth control pill: clinical trials on, 117–118; FDA approval of, 140–145; field trials on, 129–133, 138–139; financing

Progesterone, 39, 74; 19-nor, 104, 113; and pill research, 98–102, 108–114, 117; synthetic, 103, 109, 110–111

Progestins, and pill research, 113, 114, 115, 117–122, 127

Protestant denominations: current stand on birth control of, 148; early ban on birth control by, 24; resolution of, on birth control, 25, 26

Prout, Curtis, 23

Pseudo-pregnancy, 109–110, 111

Public Health Field Training Center, U.S., 128

Puerto Rico, pill field trial in, 128–133, 138–139

Puerto Rico, University of, 118, 119

Puerto Rico Family Planning Association, 128

Quinn, John R., 230

Ralls, Jack, 114

Ramcharan, Savitri, 218

Ratner, Herbert, 214

Raymond, Al, 136

Reader's Digest, 138, 155

Redbook, 155

Reed, James, *From Private Vice to Public Virtue,* 107, 184

Reid, Duncan, 200, 207

Rhythm Clinic, 43, 44, 83

Rhythm method of birth control, 26–27, 43–44, 76, 154–155; Catholic Church's stand on, 151, 190

Rice-Wray, Edris, 128, 131–132, 133, 232

Richardson, Elliot, 200

Richardson, George S., 45, 200–201

Rickettsiae, 61 and n

Riedmatten, Father de, 177

Rinman, E. Harold, 118

Rivo, Eliott, 55, 196–197

Roberts, Thomas D., 169

Robinson, Derek, 55

Rochester, University of, 98

Rock, Anna Thorndike (wife of John), 28, 29, 70, 206, 232, 233; Catholicism of, 35; children of, 20; courtship, 16–17; death of, 158; marriage, 18–23; on Miriam Menkin, 91

Rock, Ann Jane (AJ, daughter of John), 20, 21, 27–28, 36

Rock, Ann Jane Murphy (mother of John), 4, 5–6, 8

Rock, Charles (Charlie, brother of John), 6, 7, 8, 11, 22

Rock, Ellen (daughter of John), 20, 28, 35–36

Rock, Ellen (Nell, sister of John), 3, 6, 7, 17

Rock, Frank Sylvester (father of John), 4–6, 8–9, 11, 12, 22

Rock, Henry (Harry, brother of John), 6, 8

Rock, John: and birth control fight, 24, 26, 27; birth and early life of, 3, 5–8; bitterness in later life of, 193–207 *passim;* and Catholic Church's reaction to pill's approval, 146, 151, 153–173 *passim;* characterized, 44–45; children of, 20; club memberships of, 23–24; his courtship and marriage, 16–23; death of son, 30–31; early jobs of, 10–11; education of, 9–10, 11–12; on effects of heat and light on contraception, 55–56; and FDA approval of pill, 140, 142–145; Harvard chair named for, 183; Harvard's honorary degree awarded to, 184; heart attacks suffered by, 29–30, 85, 233; on human sexuality, 31–34, 42–43, 177–178; and IUDs, 185; later life of, 226–233; lectures of, 42–43, 177–180; and Katherine McCormick, 95; and Miriam Menkin, 72, 75, 89–92; on menstruation, 50–51; on odor as sexual attractant, 54–55; and papal rejection of birth control, 192; and pill field trial, 129, 130, 132–133, 139; and pill research, 98, 106–107, 109–111, 115–127 *passim;* and pill safety, 140; practice built by, 22; research of, on human reproduction, 38–40; residencies and internships of, 12–14, 17–18; and rhythm method of birth control, 26–27, 43–44; "Sex, Science and Survival," 32, 177; on tampons, 51; television appearances of, 166–167; and test-tube fertilization, 72, 75–87 *passim; The Time Has Come,* 159–166, 167, 168–169, 170, 177; Irwin C. Winter on, 135–136; his work on fertilized human eggs, 59–60, 62–71, 75; his work on infertility, 41–42, 44, 49–50, 51–53, 109–112

Rock, John (grandfather of John), 4, 6

Rock, John, Jr. (Jack, son of John), 20, 27–28, 206, 227, 233; death of, 30–31

Rock, John (uncle of John), 4–5

Rock, Martha (daughter of John), 20

Rock, Mary (Maisie, sister of John), 6

Rock, Rachel Sherman (daughter of John), 20, 29, 30, 36, 37, 66; death of her brother Jack, 30–31; on John Rock, 34

Rock-Derry Clinic, 202

Rockefeller, John D., Jr., 7